Eye Banking

Developments in Ophthalmology

Vol. 43

Series Editor

W. Behrens-Baumann Magdeburg

Eye Banking

Volume Editors

Timm Bredehorn-Mayr Halle (Saale)
Gernot I.W. Duncker Halle (Saale)
W. John Armitage Bristol

41 figures, 11 in color, and 12 tables, 2009

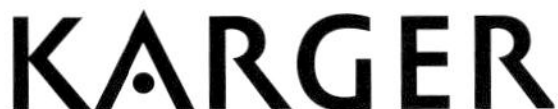

Basel · Freiburg · Paris · London · New York · Bangalore ·
Bangkok · Shanghai · Singapore · Tokyo · Sydney

T. Bredehorn-Mayr
Martin-Luther-Universität
Halle-Wittenberg
Klinikum der Medizinischen
Fakultät
Universitätsklinik und Poliklinik
für Augenheilkunde
Ernst-Grube-Str. 40
DE–06120 Halle (Saale)
(Germany)

G.I.W. Duncker
Martin-Luther-Universität
Halle-Wittenberg
Klinikum der Medizinischen
Fakultät
Universitätsklinik und
Poliklinik für Augenheilkunde
Ernst-Grube-Str. 40
DE–06120 Halle (Saale)
(Germany)

W.J. Armitage
University of Bristol
Bristol Eye Hospital
Lower Maudlin Street
Bristol BS1 2LX (UK)

Library of Congress Cataloging-in-Publication Data

Eye banking / volume editors, Timm Bredehorn-Mayr, Gernot I.W. Duncker, W. John Armitage.
p. ; cm. -- (Developments in ophthalmology, ISSN 0250-3751 ; v. 43)
Includes bibliographical references and indexes.
ISBN 978-3-8055-9124-9 (hard cover : alk. paper)
1. Eye banks. 2. Cornea--Transplantation. I. Bredehorn-Mayr, Timm. II. Duncker, Gernot. III. Armitage, W. John.
[DNLM: 1. Corneal Transplantation--Europe. 2. Eye Banks--organization & administration--Europe. W1 DE998NG v.43 2009 / WW 170 E97 2009]
RE89.E94 2009
362.17'83--dc22

2009009508

Bibliographic Indices. This publication is listed in bibliographic services, including Current Contents®.

Drug Dosage. The authors and the publisher have exerted every effort to ensure that drug selection and dosage set forth in this text are in accord with current recommendations and practice at the time of publication. However, in view of ongoing research, changes in government regulations, and the constant flow of information relating to drug therapy and drug reactions, the reader is urged to check the package insert for each drug for any change in indications and dosage and for added warnings and precautions. This is particularly important when the recommended agent is a new and/or infrequently employed drug.

www.karger.com
Printed in Switzerland on acid-free and non-aging paper (ISO 9706) by Reinhardt Druck, Basel
ISSN 0250–3751
ISBN 978–3–8055–9124–9
e-ISBN 978–3–8055–9125–6

Contents

List of Contributors

W. John Armitage, Prof., BSc, PhD
Department of Clinical Science
University of Bristol
Lower Maudlin Street
Bristol BS1 2LX (UK)

Daniel Böhringer, PD Dr. med.
Universitätsaugenklinik Freiburg
Killianstrasse 5
DE–79106 Freiburg (Germany)

A.G. Bokhorst, MD, MPH
BIS Foundation
PO Box 2304
NL–2301 CH Leiden (The Netherlands)

Vincent M. Borderie, MD, PhD
Centre Hospitalier National d'Ophtalmologie des XV–XX
28, rue de Charenton
FR–75012 Paris (France)

Timm Bredehorn-Mayr, Dr. med.
Martin-Luther-Universität Halle-Wittenberg
Klinikum der Medizinischen Fakultät
Universitätsklinik und Poliklinik für Augenheilkunde
Ernst-Grube-Str. 40
DE–06120 Halle (Saale) (Germany)

Michael Cahane, MD
EATB Ocular Council and Sheba Medical Center Eye Bank
Tel Hashomer 52621 (Israel)

Davide Camposampiero, BSc
Fondazione Banca degli Occhi del Veneto – ONLUS
Via Paccagnella n. 11 – Padiglione Rama
IT–30174 Zelarino – Venice (Italy)

Ilse Claerhout, MD, PhD
Department of Ophthalmology
Ghent University Hospital
De Pintelaan 185
BE–9000 Ghent (Belgium)

Iva Dekaris, Prof., MD, PhD
Eye Clinic 'Svjetlost'
Heinzelova 39
HR–10000 Zagreb (Croatia)

Caroline A. Dorrepaal, MD, PhD
BIS Foundation
PO Box 2304
NL–2301 CH Leiden (The Netherlands)

G.I.W. Duncker, Prof.
Martin-Luther-Universität Halle-Wittenberg
Klinikum der Medizinischen Fakultät
Universitätsklinik und Poliklinik für Augenheilkunde
Ernst-Grube-Str. 40
DE–06120 Halle (Saale) (Germany)

Niels Ehlers, Dr.
Department of Ophthalmology
Århus University Hospital
Nørrebrogade 44
DK–8000 Århus C (Denmark)

Katrin Engelmann, Prof. Dr. med.
Department of Ophthalmology
Städtisches Klinikum Chemnitz gGmbH
Flemmingstraße 2
DE–09116 Chemnitz (Germany)

Nikica Gabrić, Prof., MD, PhD
Eye Clinic 'Svjetlost'
Heinzelova 39
HR–10000 Zagreb (Croatia)

Carlo Griffoni, BSc
Fondazione Banca degli Occhi del
Veneto – ONLUS
Via Paccagnella n. 11 – Padiglione Rama
IT–30174 Zelarino – Venice (Italy)

Claudia Hauswald
Interdisciplinary Center for Medicine
Ethics and Law
Martin-Luther-University Halle-Wittenberg
DE–06108 Halle (Saale) (Germany)

Jesper Hjortdal, Dr.
Department of Ophthalmology
Århus University Hospital
Nørrebrogade 44
DK–8000 Århus C (Denmark)

Gary L. A. Jones, BSc (Econ)
Fondazione Banca degli Occhi
Administrator, European Eye Bank Association
Fondazione Banca degli Occhi del
Veneto – ONLUS
Via Paccagnella n. 11 – Padiglione Rama
IT–30174 Zelarino – Venice (Italy)

Hanneke Maas-Reijs
Cornea Bank Amsterdam,
Euro Tissue Bank
p/a NIN Meibergdreef 47
NL–1105 BA Amsterdam (The Netherlands)

P. Maier, Dr. med.
Universitätsaugenklinik Freiburg
Killianstrasse 5
DE–79106 Freiburg (Germany)

Kim Nielsen, Cand. Scient., PhD
Department of Ophthalmology
Århus University Hospital
Nørrebrogade 44
DK–8000 Århus C (Denmark)

E. Pels, PhD
Cornea Bank Amsterdam
Euro Tissue Bank
p/a NIN Meibergdreef 47
NL–1105 BA Amsterdam (The Netherlands)

Diego Ponzin, MD
Fondazione Banca degli Occhi del
Veneto – ONLUS
Via Paccagnella n. 11 – Padiglione Rama
IT–30174 Zelarino – Venice (Italy)

T. Reinhard, Prof. Dr. med.
Universitätsaugenklinik Freiburg
Killianstrasse 5
DE–79106 Freiburg (Germany)

Peter Rieck, Prof. Dr.
Cornea Bank Berlin
Department of Ophthalmology
Charité – Universitätsmedizin Berlin
Campus-Virchow-Klinikum
Augustenburger Platz 1
DE–13353 Berlin (Germany)

W.J. Rijneveld, MD
Cornea Bank Amsterdam
Euro Tissue Bank
p/a NIN Meibergdreef 47
NL–1105 BA Amsterdam (The Netherlands)

Jan Schroeter, Dr.
Cornea Bank Berlin
Department of Ophthalmology
Charité – Universitätsmedizin Berlin
Campus-Virchow-Klinikum
Augustenburger Platz 1
DE–13353 Berlin (Germany)

R. Sundmacher, Prof. Dr. med.
Universitätsaugenklinik Freiburg
Killianstrasse 5
DE–79106 Freiburg (Germany)

Mauro Toniolo, Dipl.Tech.
Fondazione Banca degli Occhi del Veneto – ONLUS
Via Paccagnella n. 11 – Padiglione Rama
IT–30174 Zelarino – Venice (Italy)

M. Töteberg-Harms
Eye Clinic
University Hospital of Zurich
CH–8032 Zurich (Switzerland)

Andrew B. Tullo, MD, FRCOphth
Manchester Eye Bank
Manchester Royal Eye Hospital
Oxford Road
M13 9WH Manchester

Monika Valtink, Dipl.-Ing. (FH)
Institute of Anatomy
Medical Faculty 'Carl Gustav Carus'
TU Dresden
Fetscherstr. 74
DE–01307 Dresden (Germany)

Jeroen van Baare, Dr., MSc
Dutch Health Care Inspectorate
Program 8 Product Safety
Wilhelmina van Pruisenweg 52
NL–2595 AN Den Haag (The Netherlands)

Preface

Corneal transplantation has been performed with increasing success for more than 100 years. In the last 20 years, standards, outcomes and developments in the field of corneal transplantation and eye banking have been discussed at the annual meetings of the European Eye Bank Association (EEBA) to share and promote good practice and guarantee a high level of safety for the recipients. The EEBA standards for donor selection and eye banking provide professional advice and guidance to eye banks and corneal surgeons.

The EU Tissues and Cells Directive (2004/23/EC) and its accompanying technical directives (Commission Directives 2006/17/EC and 2006/86/EC) came into force in 2006, setting mandatory standards for the procurement, processing, preservation, storage and distribution of human tissue for therapeutic use. This includes eye banking and the supply of ocular tissue for transplantation. The transposition of these EU directives into law is the responsibility of individual EU member states. There is still, however, a need for tissue-specific guidance from professional organizations such as the EEBA to provide more detailed advice not covered by the EU directives and, ultimately, to help improve standards for the quality and safety of tissues for human application.

This book highlights the history and development of eye banking and all significant steps including the donation, processing and distribution of corneas for transplantation. Additional contributions on the sclera, amnion and retinal pigment epithelium provide further insights into ocular surgery and the future potential for transplantation. This book contributes the essentials in eye banking activities for ophthalmologists and eye bankers as well as for regulatory and legislative authorities.

Timm Bredehorn-Mayr, Gernot I.W. Duncker, Halle (Saale)
W. John Armitage, Bristol

Bredehorn-Mayr T, Duncker GIW, Armitage WJ (eds): Eye Banking.
Dev Ophthalmol. Basel, Karger, 2009, vol 43, pp 1–14

Corneal Grafting and Banking

Niels Ehlers · Jesper Hjortdal · Kim Nielsen

Danish Eye Bank, Department of Ophthalmology, Århus University Hospital, Århus, Denmark

Abstract

Corneal transplantation was conceptualized at the end of the 18th century, but it took more than 100 years before human corneal grafting was introduced. The greatest step forward was the demonstration by Filatov that corneal tissue can be collected and used post mortem. The history of eye banking includes the development of preservation techniques. Storage in cold to minimize microbial growth and tissue disintegration was first choice but during the last 30 years this has been taken over by warm storage (organ culture) where the donor cornea proves its sterility and vitality before being transferred to the recipient. The long-term organ culture storage makes exchange between centres possible and allows for histocompatibility matching. The internationalization led to the establishing of the European Eye Bank Association but also to an increasing number of governmental regulations. Developments in years to come may lead to control of graft biomechanics and optics. This technical development tends to favour a centralization.

The Beginning of Corneal Transplantation

The replacement of the opaque cornea by an artificial transparent structure was mentioned in 1789 by de Quengsy [1] of Montpellier, France. Later (in 1824) Reisinger [2] suggested the use of an animal cornea, a procedure he named keratoplasty. During the 19th century, many animal experiments were done, and it was gradually realized that homologous tissue was necessary to avoid opacification of the graft. Human transplantations were attempted, and Zirm [3] (1906) is usually credited as the first to have performed and reported a successful grafting. It was originally believed that very fresh tissue, used in a kind of status nascendi, was important. It was therefore a most important step forward when in 1935 and 1937 Filatov [4, 5] of Odessa, Ukraine, documented the applicability of post-mortem tissue (fig. 1). This opened up to a supply of donor material, the limitations now being ethics, legislation and practical organization.

This work was presented at the Polish-Ukrainian Ophthalmological Conference in Lublin, Poland, June 29 to July 1, 2006.

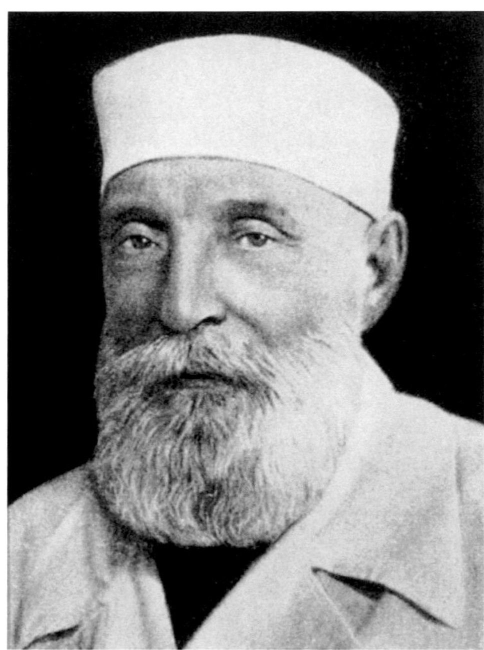

Fig. 1. F.P. Filatov.

Refinement of Surgical Technique

Over some decades in the middle of the 20th century, the corneal handling and the techniques of grafting were developed. Milestones were the routine use of a surgical microscope and the manufacturing of sufficiently delicate instruments. Every step could now be performed precisely and under direct visual control.

Early Eye Banking

Corneal preservation of the donor cornea before grafting was reported by Magitot [6] in 1912. He kept a human cornea in haemolysed blood for 8 days at 5°C before successful use as a lamellar graft. With the later observation by Filatov of the use of post-mortem tissue, the road to proper eye banking was found.

On the European continent, donor eyes were routinely obtained from hospital morgues, and the tissue was used immediately after retrieval. To overcome the practical problems in retrieving, donor tissue banks were organized, e.g. in London and New York, where donor eyes were collected and quickly redistributed.

The banking technique was originally very simple with the use of small glass bottles, in which the eyebulbs were kept under moist and cool conditions (fig. 2). Enucleation was performed as shortly after death as possible. The post-mortem time

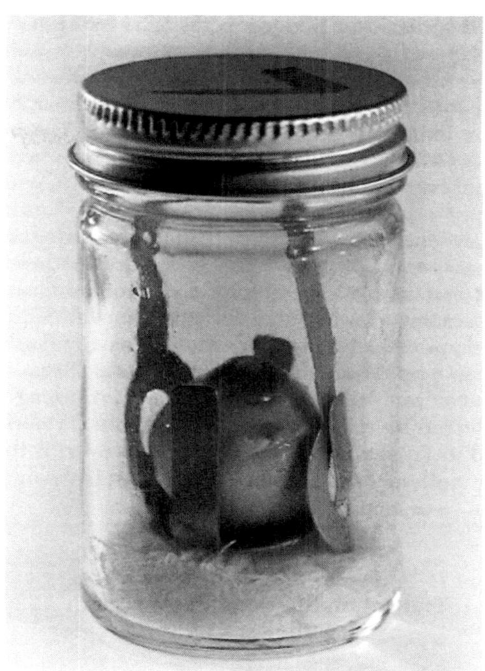

Fig. 2. Donor eye in moist chamber.

and the immediate direct appearance of the cornea were the only quality controls. The importance of a viable endothelium for a successful outcome was soon realized by Stocker [7]. Consequently corneal banking research was directed at the maintenance of viability and integrity of this layer.

Current Preservation Techniques

Several methods for corneal preservation are currently in use throughout the world. None of these techniques is ideal but each provides benefits and disadvantages. The main differences regard storage temperature, medium composition and presence of an osmotic agent to prevent stromal swelling. In the following paragraphs the moist chamber storage, the cold medium storage and the cryopreservation techniques will be briefly presented before turning to a more detailed discussion of the organ culture methods.

Moist Chamber

The entire globe or the excised cornea may be kept under moist and cool conditions for hours and up to 1–2 days. It is the traditional method when donor corneas are collected at the hospital morgue and used the same day. The technique is simple and requires almost no equipment. It is therefore still in use in some locations. With access to fresh donor material, the results are excellent. However, aspects such as microbiological contamination, transmission of donor diseases and histocompatibility are neglected. Today, therefore, the method is replaced by preservation of the isolated cornea in various solutions kept at 4°C (cold storage) or at body temperature (30–37°C, organ culture conditions).

Cold Storage

This technique of storage at 4°C was developed by McCarey and Kaufman [8] in 1974 using a standard culture medium (TC-199) supplemented with antibiotics and dextran as antiswelling agent. Due to the low temperature, the metabolism of the cornea is reduced to a minimum but viability is not demonstrated, infection not disclosed and the cornea can only be maintained for days (up to 7–10 days).

Cryopreservation

For years the establishment of a bank of cryopreserved donor corneas was considered a goal. The donor corneas should be waiting for the patients. This idea was based on reports on successful use of frozen and thawed human tissue [9, 10], and for some time it was thought that cryopreservation could provide the solution to the cornea banking problems. In 1965, Capella et al. [11] improved the technique with dimethylsulphoxide as cryoprotectant. This method was clinically useful but its complexity, e.g. the requirement of very fresh tissue to be frozen, prevented a widespread use. In 1981, Sperling [12] developed a technique with cryopreservation of tissue at first kept under organ culture conditions, then frozen. After thawing the tissue was once again organ cultured to prove its vitality. The clinical results with this cryopreservation procedure were reported in 1982 [13]. After 1 year 71% clear grafts were found, and even after 12 years [14] the graft survival was 58%.

The conclusion to be drawn is that cryopreservation can be done and a bank of frozen tissue could be established, but the technique would be very demanding. Still, however, research is going on and the possibility of undercooling, i.e. maintenance of the tissue at a temperature below zero but without crystallization in the tissue, is another not yet fully explored possibility [15].

Organ Culture

The organ culture technique is based on the idea of a long-term preservation of the isolated human cornea under simulated physiological conditions. The main advantage of such an approach is that the donor cornea can prove its viability and sterility in the culture flask rather than failing in the patient's eye. So-called primary graft failures do not occur or are extremely rare.

The organ culture technique was introduced in the 1970s [16, 17] and brought to Europe by Sperling, who in the following years modified and developed the technique into clinical routine (fig. 3). The technique was later reintroduced in the USA as the 'Minnesota system' [18, 19]. Extensive research and long-term clinical use in Europe document the safety of the organ culture method. The organ culture method is today the method of choice in Western Europe.

Eye Banking Procedures in Denmark

The number of corneas required for grafting in Denmark is less than 500/year. All corneas in the country are supplied by one eye bank, the Danish Eye Bank, at Århus University Hospital. Since 1979 exclusively organ-cultured corneas have been used.

After laboratory development of the technique [20] (fig. 4–7) and quality documentation by comparison to fresh material [21] (fig. 8), the routine procedure described below was established.

Retrieval and Primary Evaluation

Retrieval of donor tissue is done by specially trained technicians removing the whole globe. Simultaneously a blood sample is taken. The post-mortem time is not critical. The eyebulbs and the blood samples are transported to the eye bank and stored in a refrigerator.

Primary evaluation of the donor cornea is done by visual inspection followed by 30 s of rinsing in tap water. The cornea is excised with a scleral rim and the endothelium inspected under an ordinary light microsope after trypan blue staining. The cells are outlined by the temporary swelling of the intercellular spaces [22]. The cornea is then suspended by a suture in a culture bottle with minimal essential medium containing 10% fetal calf serum.

Organ Culture and Sterility Checks

The cornea is kept in the closed bottle at 31°C until 1 day before use.

Under sterile conditions, a sample of the medium is withdrawn after 1–2 weeks and examined at the microbiological laboratory for bacterial and fungal contamination. The tissue is in quarantine until negative test results are received. The 'banking time' is usually 2–4 weeks but may, after exchange of medium, be extended to 7 weeks [23] and probably even longer.

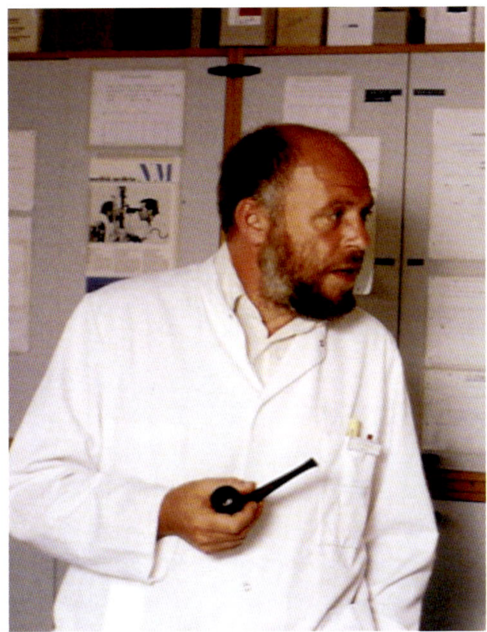

Fig. 3. S. Sperling developed the organ culture technique for clinical use.

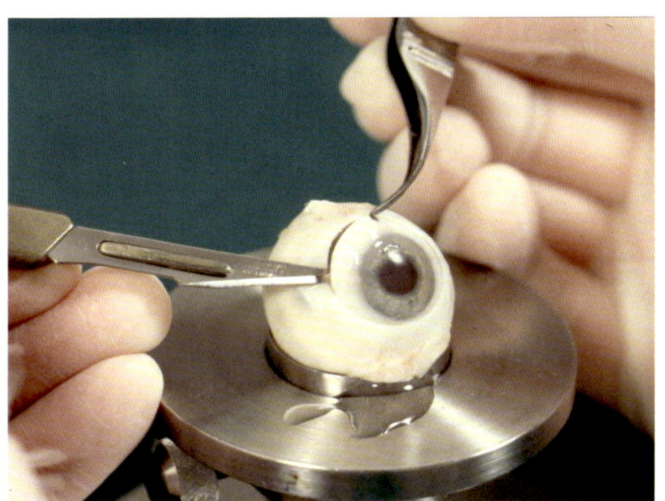

Fig. 4. Preparation of a cornea with a scleral rim.

Preparation for Clinical Use

On the day prior to use, the medium is inspected for turbidity. If the medium is clear, the bottle is opened in a laminar flow bench. The endothelium is inspected after staining and cell border swelling. Cell density is estimated but not routinely quantitated. The cornea is then transferred to new medium with addition of 5% dextran to deswell the stroma.

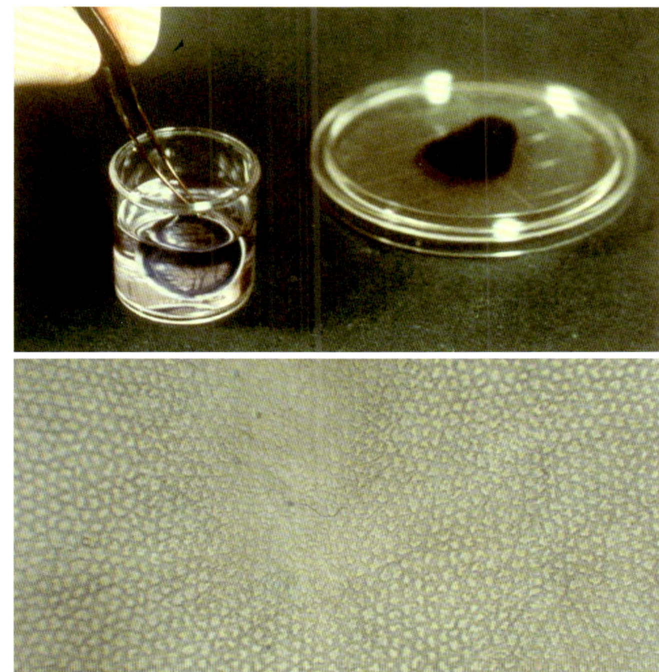

Fig. 5. Staining endothelium with trypan blue.

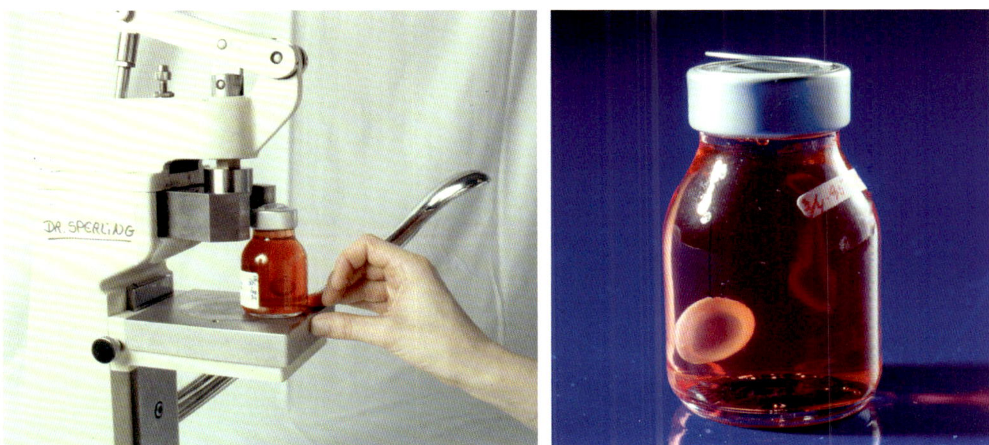

Fig. 6. Closed-system preparation.

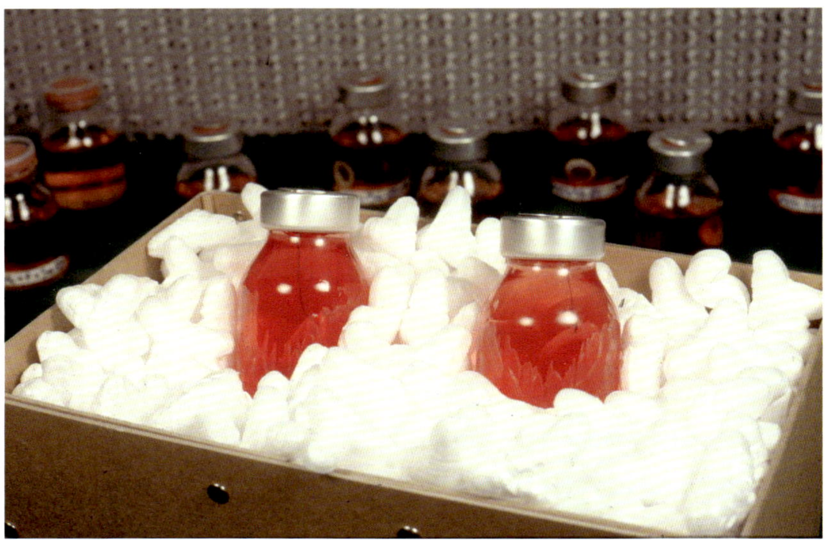

Fig. 7. Donor corneas packed for shipping.

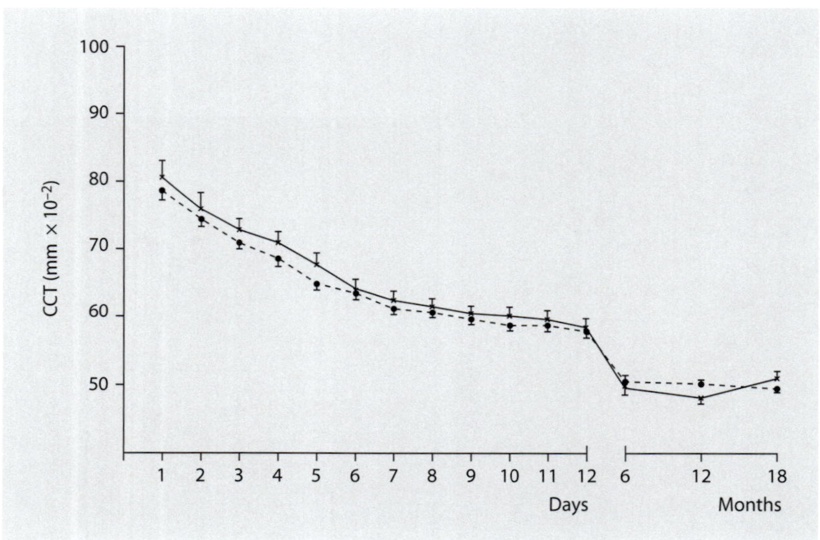

Fig. 8. No difference in immediate and late deswelling of fresh and organ-cultured corneas. CCT = Central corneal thickness.

For transportation, the bottle is packed in a shock-absorbing box and sent by ordinary surface mail to the receiver.

Documentation

The cornea is labelled for identification.

Modern-Day Results

Today results from keratoplasty are generally satisfactory. The success rate depends upon the quality of the donor tissue and the condition of the recipient corneal bed.

Vascularization and earlier graft rejection have a negative influence. In non-risk cases, the success rate is between 90 and 100%. In risk cases, the success rate falls to 50% or less [21] (fig. 9).

These percentages refer to a limited observation time. Even if the risk of rejection decreases with time, endothelial rejection can still occur after many years. A recently observed rejection in a keratoconus patient occurred after 18 years and was reversed by steroid treatment.

In biology the concept of compatibility is recognized. Organs are successfully exchanged between identical twins. The compatibility is described by the complex HLA system comprising at least 2 classes (I and II) that are of importance. Most clinical studies find histocompatibility to be of importance for the outcome.

What is however still an unsettled question is the logistics of handling compatibility and corneal grafting.

With a given HLA genotype and knowledge of the prevalence of the different HLA genes, an expected waiting time for a compatible donor can be calculated [24]. This must be compared to the patient's age and life expectancy. Evidently, the more donors, the shorter the waiting time. Therefore exchange of tissue between banks (and countries) becomes an interesting issue. This situation was in fact recognized 30 years ago. The need for a collaboration between eye banks has been a stimulus for creation of an eye bank association.

The European Eye Bank Association

The first meeting, in what turned out to be the European Eye Bank Association (EEBA), was held in Århus, Denmark, in 1989. From that meeting, it was clear that there was a need to coordinate our efforts to organize and develop the eye bank concept, mainly following the procedures for organ culture. Since then annual meetings have been held, and the name EEBA was suggested by Andrew Tullo, Manchester,

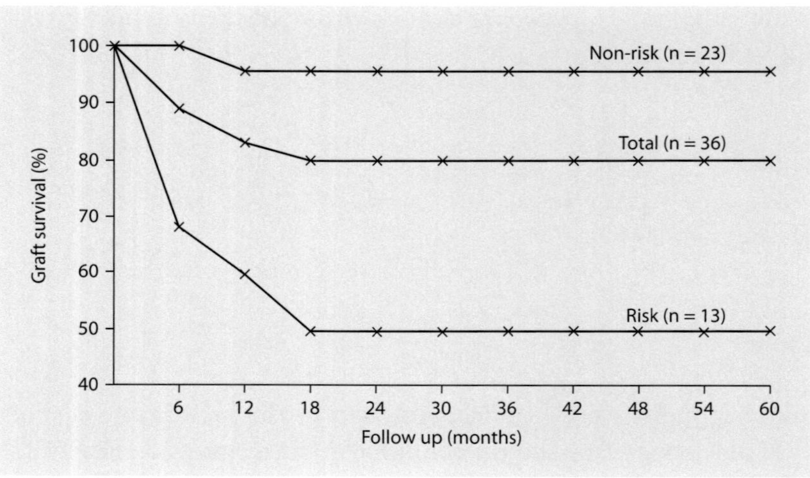

Fig. 9. Success rate of grafting: 5-year graft survival.

UK. The EEBA has now grown to include (in 2006) 79 member eye banks. The number of corneas retrieved and processed in 2005 was almost 35,000. The majority of corneas passed through organ culture but a substantial number is still used after cold storage.

Another purpose of the EEBA was to set standards for eye banking. At the meetings the rules, recommendations etc. were discussed. The viewpoints of the EEBA were gradually formulated, and today an annual directory is published [25] (fig. 10).

European Union Regulations

The entire area of organ donation, retrieval and handling of organs and tissues has become an issue of greatest interest. One driving force was the fear of transferring diseases to the recipients.

Legislations regulating transplantation of corneal tissue have varied considerably between national states. In some countries, the cornea has been considered a piece of tissue, in other countries it has been looked upon as an organ. The Directive 2004/23/EC of the European Parliament and of the Council of March 31, 2004, is within the near future going to set the standards of quality and safety for the donation, procurement, testing, processing, preservation, storage and distribution of human tissues and cells – including corneal tissue.

The main objective of the directive is to ensure the quality and safety of tissue transplantations, particularly in order to prevent transmission of diseases. The directive is followed by two appendices specifically defining (1) certain technical requirements

1989 Århus
1990 Bristol
1991 Noordwijk
1992 Wien
1993 Bern
1994 Palma de Mallorca
1995 Budapest
1996 Besançon
1997 Venezia
1998 Aachen
1999 Zagreb
2000 Århus
2001 Örebro
2002 Paris
2003 Brussels
2004 Barcelona
2005 Halle
2006 Venezia
EEBA
EUROPEAN
EYE BANK
ASSOCIATION

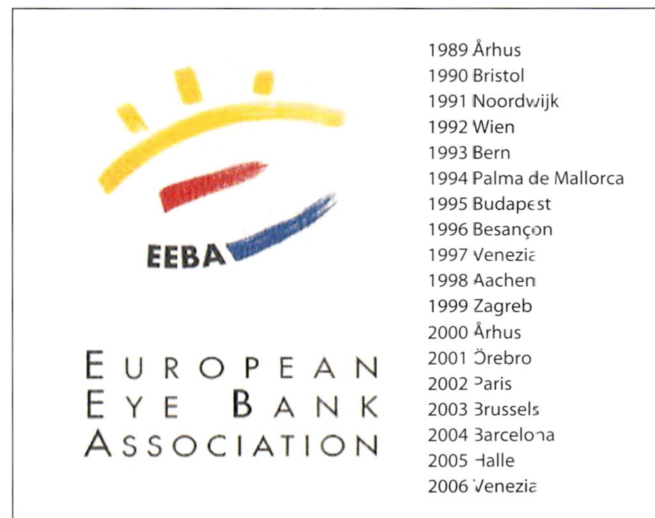

Fig. 10. EEBA logo and meetings.

for the donation, procurement and testing of human tissues and cells (Commission Directive 2006/17/EC) and (2) technical requirements for the coding, processing, preservation, storage and distribution of human tissues and cells, now published as Commission Directive 2006/86/EC. The net effect of these directives which will later be implemented in the legislation of the national states will ensure a certain minimal standard also of corneal donor tissue within Europe. On the other hand, the directives will impose a significant administrative burden on each of the many European corneal banks.

Future Developments in Eye Banking

In most eye banks, the organ culture technique has not been modified considerably throughout the last 20 years. Fetal calf serum is used in most banks to enrich the tissue-preserving properties of the culture medium. Due to fear of prion transmission from cattle to human recipients of corneal tissue potentially leading to variant Creutzfeldt-Jakob disease, there has been significant interest in developing a fully synthetic and defined culture medium for corneal organ culture [26–28]. Such media have now been developed, and prospective experiments are ongoing to optimize medium composition.

Corneal rejection directed towards the endothelial cells of the grafted tissue remains one of the main causes of graft failure. Histocompatibility between host and recipient with respect to class II [29, 30] (fig. 11) and/or class I [31] improves graft prognosis in high-risk cases and maybe also in normal-risk cases after keratoplasty [32]. The waiting time to find a good match between donor and recipient depends on

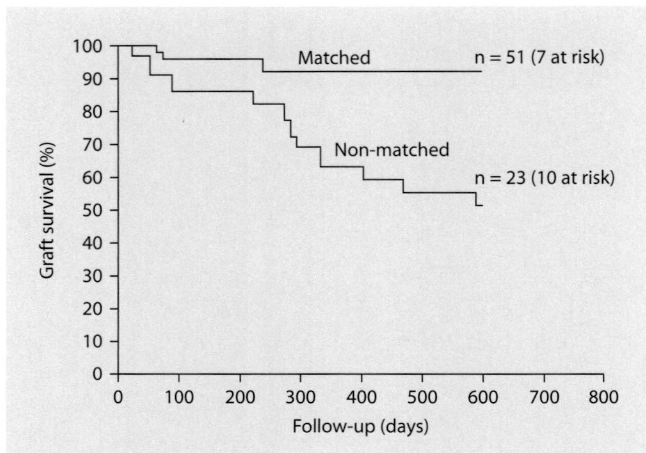

Fig. 11. Survival of HLA-matched and non-matched grafts. $\chi^2 = 8.701$; $2p = 0.0032$.

the number of donor corneas available and tested and on the frequency of the recipient tissue type (and subtypes) in the donor population. With a small supply of donor tissue, it may take years to find an optimal match. Further international collaboration between eye banks may in the future increase the pool of donors and shorten the waiting time.

After establishing methods for the isolation and in vitro cultivation of human corneal endothelial cells, isolated transplantation of endothelial cells may be an alternative therapeutic option [33]. With the techniques of modern molecular biology, it may be assumed that cultured endothelial cells with low expression of histocompatibility antigens can be manufactured – or even that the recipient's own endothelial cells can be made to proliferate in vitro and be autotransplanted back to the patient. This latter approach seems to be possible today for epithelial cells [34].

Development of a purely synthetic cornea would be the ultimate way to overcome the relative lack of suitable donor tissue and the ever more important burden of administrative work related to transplantation of human tissue. Today, promising results from a recent study suggest that lamellar corneal grafts may be produced synthetically [35].

Development of a purely synthetic cornea is also the target for international research programmes (Centres nationaux de la recherche scientifique).

Graft Optics

With an established surgical and banking technique, another problem becomes evident. Grafted corneas are only occasionally spherical. Some degree of astigmatism is the rule. Average values in clinical series are around 2–4 dpt. In addition higher-order optical aberrations often compromise the visual result. This optical problem is approached from two sides. Laser reshapening of the surface after suture removal would seem to be a manageable solution. Results may be good but another time-consuming surgical procedure rarely excites the patient. Therefore attempts are made to avoid astigmatism, e.g. by laser excision of the graft and recipient cornea (non-mechanical technique), a refined suture technique or mechanical stabilization by metal or plastic inlays, or increasing the tissue stiffness by molecular cross-linking.

Development of new lamellar surgical techniques for changing either the anterior or posterior part of the cornea is promising. Anterior lamellar grafting is used in keratoconus and other stromal dystrophies with the advantage of avoiding transplantation of endothelial cells [36]. Posterior lamellar grafting can be used in Fuchs' dystrophy or secondary bullous keratopathy. In the more recent techniques, the so-called Descemet's stripping endothelial keratoplasty, removal of the dysfunctioning endothelium and underlying Descemet's membrane, is performed through a peripheral 5-mm corneal incision [37]. The advantage is faster visual recovery, less astigmatism and a more stable eye compared with the traditional penetrating keratoplasty procedure.

References

1 Pellier de Quengsy G: Précis au cours d'operations sur la chirurgie des yeux. Paris, Didot, 1789.

2 Reisinger FR: Die Keratoplastik, ein Versuch zur Erweiterung der Augenheilkunde. Bayer Ann 1824;I:207.

3 Zirm E: Eine erfolgreiche totale Keratoplastik. Arch Ophthalmol 1906;64:580–593.

4 Filatov VP: Transplantation of the cornea. Arch Ophthalmol 1935;13:321–347.

5 Filatov VP: Transplantation of the cornea from preserved cadavers' eyes. Lancet 1937;i:1395–1397.

6 Magitot A: Transplantation of the human cornea previously preserved in an antiseptic fluid. JAMA 1912;59:18–21.

7 Stocker FW: The endothelium of the cornea and its clinical implications. Trans Am Ophthalmol Soc 1953;51:669–786.

8 McCarey BE, Kaufman HE: Improved corneal storage. Invest Opthalmol 1974;13:165–173.

9 Eastcott HHG, Gross AG, Leigh AG, North DP: Preservation of corneal graft by freezing. Lancet 1954;i:237–244.

10 Müller FO, Smith AU: Some experiments on grafting frozen corneal tissue in rabbits. Exp Eye Res 1963;2:237–246.

11 Capella JA, Kaufman HE, Robbins JE: Preservation of viable corneal tissue. Arch Ophthalmol 1965;74: 669–673.

12 Sperling S: Cryopreservation of human cadaver corneas regenerated at 31°C in a modified tissue culture medium. Acta Ophthalmol Copenh 1981;59: 142–148.

13 Ehlers N, Sperling S, Olsen T: Post-operative thickness and endothelial cell density in cultivated, cryopreserved human corneal grafts. Acta Opthalmol Copenh 1982;60:935–944.

14 Erdmann L, Ehlers N: Long-term results with organ cultured, cryopreserved human corneal grafts: reexamination of 17 patients. Acta Ophthalmol Copenh 1993;71:703–706.

15 Rich SJ, Armitage WJ: Corneal tolerance of vitrifiable concentrations of glycerol. Cryobiology 1992; 29:153–164.

16 Summerlin WT, Miller GE, Harris JE, Good RA: The organ-cultured cornea: an in vitro study. Invest Ophthalmol 1973;12:176–180.

17 Bourne WM, Doughman DJ, Lindstrom RL: Organ-cultured corneal endothelium in vivo. Arch Ophthalmol 1977;95:1818–1819.

18 Lindstrom RL, Doughman DJ, Skelnik DL, Mindrup EA: Minnesota system corneal preservation. Dev Ophthalmol 1985;11:37–43.
19 Lindstrom RL, Doughman DJ, Skelnik DL, Mindrup EA: Minnesota system corneal preservation. Br J Ophthalmol 1986;70:47–54.
20 Sperling S: Human corneal endothelium in organ culture: the influence of temperature and medium of incubation. Acta Ophthalmol Copenh 1979;57:269–276.
21 Andersen J, Ehlers N: Corneal transplantation using long-term cultured material. Acta Ophthalmol Copenh 1986;64:93–96.
22 Sperling S: Early morphological changes in organ cultured human corneal endothelium. Acta Ophthalmol Copenh 1978;56:785–792.
23 Ehlers H, Ehlers N, Hjortdal JØ: Corneal transplantation with donor tissue kept in organ culture for 7 weeks. Acta Ophthalmol Copenh 1999;77:277–278.
24 Sundmacher R (ed): Adequate HLA Matching in Keratoplasty. Dev Ophthalmol. Basel, Karger, vol 36.
25 EEBA: Directory of European Cornea Bank Association, ed 14. Venezia Mestre, EEBA, 2006.
26 Moller-Pedersen T, Hartmann U, Ehlers N, Engelmann K: Evaluation of potential organ culture media for eye banking using human donor corneas. Br J Ophthalmol 2001;85:1075–1079.
27 Moller-Pedersen T, Hartmann U, Ehlers N, Engelmann K: Evaluation of potential organ culture media for eye banking using a human corneal endothelial cell growth assay. Graefes Arch Clin Exp Ophthalmol 2001;239:778–782.
28 Hempel B, Bednarz J, Engelmann K: Use of a serum-free medium for long-term storage of human corneas: influence on endothelial cell density and corneal metabolism. Graefes Arch Clin Exp Ophthalmol 2001;239:801–805.
29 Baggesen K, Lamm LU, Ehlers N: Effect of HLA-DR/RFLP matching in complicated corneal transplantations. ClinTransplant 1990;21:197–201.
30 Baggesen K, Lamm LU, Ehlers N: Significant effect of high-resolution HLA-DRB1 matching in high-risk corneal transplantation. Transplantation 1996;62:1273–1277.
31 Vail A, Gore SM, Bradley BA, Easty DLl, Rogers CA, Armitage WJ: Conclusions of the corneal transplant follow-up study: collaborating surgeons. Br J Ophthalmol 1997;81:631–636.
32 Reinhard T, Bohringer D, Enczmann J, Kogler G, Mayweg S, Wernet P, Sundmacher R: Improvement of graft prognosis in penetrating normal-risk keratoplasty by HLA class I and II matching. Eye 2004;18:269–277.
33 Engelmann K, Bednarz J, Valtink M: Prospects for endothelial transplantation. Exp Eye Res 2004;78:573–578.
34 Rama P, Bonini S, Lambiase A, Golisano O, Paterna P, De Luca M, Pellegrini G: Autologous fibrin-cultured limbal stem cells permanently restore the corneal surface of patients with total limbal stem cell deficiency. Transplantation 2001;72:1478–1485.
35 Liu Y, Gan L, Carlsson DJ, Fagerholm P, Lagali N, Watsky MA, Munger R, Hodge WG, Priest D, Griffith M: A simple, cross-linked collagen tissue substitute for corneal implantation. Invest Ophthalmol Vis Sci 2006;47:1869–1875.
36 Busin M, Zambianchi L, Arffa RC: Microkeratome-assisted lamellar keratoplasty for the surgical treatment of keratoconus. Ophthalmology 2005;112:987–997.
37 Price FWJ, Price MO: Descemet's stripping with endothelial keratoplasty in 200 eyes: early challenges and techniques to enhance donor adherence. J Cataract Refract Surg 2006;32:411–418.

Niels Ehlers
Department of Ophthalmology, Århus University Hospital
Nørrebrogade 44
DK–8000 Århus C (Denmark)
Tel. +45 89 49 32 22, Fax +45 86 12 16 53, E-Mail neh@tdcadsl.dk

Bredehorn-Mayr T, Duncker GIW, Armitage WJ (eds): Eye Banking.
Dev Ophthalmol. Basel, Karger, 2009, vol 43, pp 15–21

European Eye Bank Association

Gary L.A. Jones[a] · Diego Ponzin[a] · Elisabeth Pels[b] · Hanneke Maas[b] · Andrew B. Tullo[c] · Ilse Claerhout[d]

[a]Fondazione Banca degli Occhi del Veneto, Venice, Italy; [b]Cornea Bank Amsterdam, Euro Tissue Bank, Amsterdam, The Netherlands; [c]Manchester Eye Bank, Manchester Royal Eye Hospital, Manchester, UK; [d]Central Tissue Bank, Ghent University Hospital, Ghent, Belgium

Abstract

Background: The European Eye Bank Association (EEBA) is a technical-scientific organization for eye banks. Founded in 1989 with the simple objective of sharing information on eye banking, the Association is today the leading pan-national association in Europe dedicated to the advancement of eye banking and an authoritative reference point for eye banks which work according to quality standards. **Methods:** The Association establishes and maintains an agreed set of medical and technical standards, promotes the collection of data on eye bank activities and processes, provides opportunities for the discussion of all aspects of eye banking practice, including eye donor selection and procurement, relevant research and development, education and training in eye banking, and maintains linkage with national and international corneal transplant communities and relevant bodies. **Results:** The recent introduction of a more structured and focused committee, a permanent secretariat, the development of a website has enabled the Association to establish closer links and collaborative activities with key regulatory bodies and to provide a more constant exchange of clinical, scientific and technical ideas and best practice with fellow professionals by means of its annual meetings, the EEBA directory and website, and a regular newsletter. **Conclusion:** The EEBA is a scientific organization committed to defining minimum standards and to encouraging eye banks to maintain the highest possible standards for quality and safety. Through its annual meetings, and the collection and exchange of detailed information from member eye banks, the Association can rightly claim to speak with a confident and representative voice on eye banking in Europe.

The European Eye Bank Association (EEBA) is a technical-scientific organization comprising individual members from over 80 eye banks located in some 22 European countries. Founded with the simple objective of sharing information on eye banking, the Association is today the leading pan-national association in Europe dedicated to eye banking and an authoritative reference point for eye banks which work according to quality standards.

The Association has been formed for the advancement of eye banking (tissues and cells for treatment of eye diseases) in Europe to:

- contribute to the development and maintenance of standards;
- establish and maintain an agreed set of EEBA standards;
- promote data collection on graft outcome in order to validate techniques;
- facilitate the interchange of information between banks;
- provide opportunities for the discussion of all aspects of practice including eye donor selection and procurement;
- encourage relevant research and development;
- provide informed comment to external agencies;
- foster education and training;
- maintain national and international links with corneal transplant communities and relevant bodies;
- make knowledge in the field of eye banking available to any person for the general good of society.

Background

The first meeting of the EEBA took place in Århus, Denmark, in 1989. The handful of people present, invited by Prof. Niels Ehlers, could not have known how the organization would develop, only that there was much to learn and share about eye banking. This open-minded approach is surely one of the reasons why the EEBA is today a successful organization.

Whilst relative informality has always been a key characteristic of the EEBA, recent developments in the regulation of tissue banking in EU member states [1–3], have meant that the Association has needed to revise its objectives, rules and finances. Therefore, in September 2002, the EEBA Committee met for the first time between annual meetings to be briefed on and discuss new developments prior to the regular annual meeting.

At that time it was decided that a part-time secretariat would be established and hosted at the Veneto Eye Bank Foundation in Venice (Italy). In addition, the elected members of the EEBA Committee were clearly defined as the President, Vice-President, Secretary, Treasurer, the Technical Representative and 7 Region Officers, all with voting rights and terms of office of 3 years. Additionally, the Directory Supervisor, the Chair of the Medical Special Interest Group (SIG), the Website Manager, the organizer of the next annual meeting and the organizer of the previous year's annual meeting were confirmed as ex officio members of the Committee.

Standards

The EEBA maintains a set of recommendations ('Agreements on minimum standards') [4] relating to the medical assessment of donors and contra-indications to

Table 1. Number of responding eye banks (biennial data shown)

	1991	1993	1995	1997	1999	2001	2003	2005	2007
Banks	19	34	50	70	75	65	83	54	66
Countries	11	14	22	22	22	21	20	19	19
Corneas processed	11,530	18,594	22,722	27,713	32,497	36,567	41,709	28,534	32,080

transplantation of ocular tissues. These standards are subjected to a formal annual review by the Medical SIG but may be reviewed more frequently should the need arise. The review takes into account current professional guidance [5] and clinical practice, as well as relevant national and international regulations. Recommendations from the Medical SIG for amendments and/or additions in the light of changing standards and practices are put to the EEBA Committee for approval.

In addition, the EEBA has established a series of 'Technical guidelines for ocular tissues' [6] which define the minimally accepted standards of quality and safety for the procurement, retrieval, processing, storage and evaluation of corneal and scleral tissue for transplantation. These standards are subject to periodic review by the Technical SIG, and any proposals for changes must be submitted to the EEBA Committee for approval.

Changes to the EEBA standards approved by the Committee must be agreed by members at a business meeting of the Association. At least 21 members must be present and two thirds of those voting must be in favour before any change is fully implemented.

Directory

Details concerning technical aspects of European eye banks, along with a yearly overview of the activities of those banks, have been collected and presented since 1991 in the form of an annual directory, published in time for the annual meeting [7–9]. Unfortunately, not all banks submit annual data, and therefore some analyses do not include all the statistics from the total number of banks present in Europe (table 1).

Table 2 shows the differently sized banks, arbitrarily divided according to their activity, expressed as number of corneas issued per year.

The decrease in the percentage of corneas issued for transplantation, over the period 1991–2007, can be attributed to the more stringent quality and safety standards and regulations with regard to donor screening, serological and microbiological testing and corneal evaluation criteria (e.g. minimal endothelial cell density accepted; table 3).

Table 2. Number of differently sized banks

Corneas issued per year	1991	1993	1995	1997	1999	2001	2003	2005	2007
<50	3	4	10	11	11	4	5	5	4
50–100	4	7	7	18	20	16	19	13	15
100–500	8	17	21	29	33	37	50	26	38
500–1,000	2	4	7	7	4	5	6	7	4
>1,000	2	2	3	3	4	4	4	3	4

Table 3. Percentage of corneas discarded/unsuitable for transplantation

	1991	1993	1995	1997	1999	2001	2003	2005	2007
Corneas unsuitable for transplantation	39	41	39	42	45	48	48	44	47
Positive serology (including inadequate blood samples or dubious or incomplete test results)	3.8	5.4	5.4	7.5	6.1	6.2	9.1	7.6	11.9
Contamination rates (organ culture)	2.1	3.1	3.5	3.1	3.4	3.8	4.4	4.1	3.4

Organ culture remains the preferred routine storage method in Europe. In 2007, organ culture was used by 46 banks (70%), hypothermic storage by 13 banks (20%) and 7 banks used both methods together (10%).

The minimum criteria for donor selection are those laid down by the EEBA, although many member eye banks apply additional donor criteria and contra-indications (table 4).

The Association is committed to encouraging banks to produce standard operating procedures and to put into action a quality management system, based on the principles of good medical practice and in accordance with the requirements laid down by national authorities responsible for the accreditation, designation, authorization and licensing of tissue establishments in compliance with the EU directive (table 5).

Membership

Individuals who wish to become EEBA members will be expected to share the aims of the Association and abide by the EEBA standards. Membership is on an individual

Table 4. Criteria for acceptance and contra-indications additional to those of the EEBA

	Number of banks
Minimum age (3 months to 18 years)	46
Maximum age (65–93 years)	31
Maximum post-mortem interval to enucleation/excision	39
Medical contra-indications	
Cancer	12
Tuberculosis	18
Parkinson's disease	40
Polycythaemia vera	12
Intoxication	18
Chemotherapy	13
Cachexia	10
Anorexia	9
Guillain-Barré syndrome	22
Ocular contra-indications	
Cataract surgery	25
Ocular melanoma in posterior part of the eye	50

Table 5. Quality management

	2003	2007
Standard operating procedures	60 (7)	58 (4)
Quality manual	50 (10)	49 (8)
ISO 9001:2000 certification	1	15
EBAA certification	1	1
Other certification	2	19
Quality and technical summary	53 (5)	52 (9)

Figures in parentheses indicate those in preparation. EBAA = Eye Bank Association of America.

basis (ordinary member), and each member is required to pay an annual subscription fee in order to receive the following benefits:

- a registration fee discount for the EEBA annual meeting;
- inclusion in the EEBA directory (provided that data are delivered in time);
- a personal copy of the EEBA newsletter;
- access to training opportunities;
- right of entry to the members-only section of the website.

One ordinary member from each eye bank is identified as the corresponding member who assumes the responsibility of returning data annually in order to compile the directory. Failure to return data by the specified deadline may result in that particular eye bank not being listed in the directory.

Any ordinary member may upon retirement request to become a retired member. Retired members need not pay the annual subscription, but will have all of the privileges of ordinary membership.

Any member may recommend for honorary membership any person of distinction who has contributed outstandingly to the aims of the Association. Proposals for honorary membership will be discussed and voted on by the Committee. Honorary members need not pay the annual subscription but will have all of the privileges of ordinary membership.

The Committee may invite the President-Chair of non-European eye banking organizations to become an invited member for the duration of his/her post. Invited members need not pay the annual subscription but will have all of the privileges of ordinary membership and may at the discretion of the Committee receive financial support in attending the annual or committee meeting.

Successes

The evolving regulatory landscape in the field of tissues and cells, in particular the implementation of the European directive on setting standards of quality and safety for the donation, procurement, testing, processing, storage and distribution of human tissues and cells (Directive 2004/23/EC) and associated technical directives, meant that the EEBA needed to change in order to provide more effective and timely information and advice to its members. The introduction of a more structured and focused committee, a permanent secretariat and a dedicated website has enabled the Association to meet the challenges put before it. It has built closer links and collaborative activities with key regulatory bodies, and provided a more constant exchange of clinical, scientific and technical ideas and best practice with fellow professionals by means of its annual meetings, the EEBA directory and the EEBA website, along with the instigation of a regular newsletter.

The EEBA has helped to make eye banking in Europe more efficient and safer and has established its standing as a recognized and respected pan-European association, acknowledged by the World Health Organization WHO), the European Commission, the European Association of Tissue Banks and the Eye Bank Association of America. In addition, the Association has been consulted for its expert opinion by the European Commission Health and Consumer Protection Directorate-General (Directorate C – public health and risk assessment, C6 – health measures) and by the WHO Expert Committee on Biological Standardization, and invited to attend the Council of Europe meeting of the Group of Specialists on quality assurance for organs, tissues and cells (SP-S-QA Committee).

Conclusions

The Association's annual meetings over 20 years, and the collection and exchange of detailed information from member eye banks, amount to a significant track record such that the EEBA can rightly claim to speak with a confident voice on eye banking in Europe. As a scientific group, the EEBA remains committed to defining and upholding minimum standards and to encouraging banks to produce standard operating procedures as required by the relevant authorities in each country.

The continued support of its membership is essential in maintaining and enhancing the Association's strong reputation, and all medical, scientific and technical colleagues working in the field of eye banking (tissues and cells for treatment of eye diseases) are invited to join the Association (see www.europeaneyebanks.org for details).

References

1 Directive 2004/23/EC of the European Parliament and of the Council of March 31, 2004, on setting standards of quality and safety for the donation, procurement, testing, processing, preservation, storage and distribution of human tissues and cells. Official Journal of the European Union, L102/48, 7 April 2004.

2 Commission Directive 2006/17/EC of February 8, 2006, implementing Directive 2004/23/EC of the European Parliament and of the Council as regards certain technical requirements for the donation, procurement and testing of human tissues and cells. Official Journal of the European Union, L38/40, 9 February 2006.

3 Commission Directive 2006/86/EC implementing Directive 2004/23/EC of the European Parliament and of the Council as regards traceability requirements, notification of serious adverse reactions and events and certain technical requirements for the coding, processing, preservation, storage and distribution of human tissues and cells. Official Journal of the European Union, L294/32, 25 October 2006.

4 European Eye Bank Association: Agreements on minimum standards. April 2008.

5 Eye Bank Association of America: Medical standards. November 2008.

6 European Eye Bank Association: Technical guidelines for ocular tissues. January 2009.

7 European Eye Bank Association: Directory, ed 1, 1991; ed 17, 2009.

8 Maas-Reijs H, Pels E, Tullo AB: Eye banking in Europe. Acta Ophthalmol Scand 1997;75:541–543.

9 Pels E, Claerhout I, Maas-Reijs H, Tullo AB: Fifteen years of Eye banking in Europe. Proceedings of the 19th Annual EEBA Meeting, Bratislava, January 2007.

Gary Jones
International Coordinator
Fondazione Banca degli Occhi del Veneto – ONLUS
Administrator
European Eye Bank Association
Via Paccagnella n. 11 – Padiglione Rama
IT–30174 Zelarino – Venice (Italy)
Tel. +39 041 9656422, Fax +39 041 9656421, E-Mail admin@europeaneyebanks.org

Bredehorn-Mayr T, Duncker GIW, Armitage WJ (eds): Eye Banking.
Dev Ophthalmol. Basel, Karger, 2009, vol 43, pp 22–30

Donor Selection, Retrieval and Preparation of Donor Tissue

Donor Selection

Vincent M. Borderie

Centre Hospitalier National d'Ophtalmologie des XV–XX, Paris, France

Abstract

Corneal transplantation safety is widely dependent on clinical donor selection. Donor-to-host transmission of rabies and Creutzfeldt-Jakob disease is well established, and it is lethal for the recipient. Taking into consideration this latter figure, contraindications to ocular tissue transplantation include not only rabies, contact with rabies virus, spongiform encephalitis, family history of spongiform encephalitis, recipients of human pituitary-derived hormones before 1987, surgery using dura mater and brain/spinal surgery before 1992, but also CNS diseases of unknown etiology or those with unknown risk of transmission. It has been established that hepatitis B virus and herpes simplex virus can be transmitted by corneal transplantation, and both diseases are contraindications to transplantation. HIV infection, syphilis, hepatitis C, hepatitis A, tuberculosis, HTLV-1 and -2 infection, active leprosy, active typhoid, smallpox and active malaria are also contraindications to ocular tissue transplantation even if no evidence of donor-to-recipient transmission has been demonstrated. A history of corneal refractive surgery in the donor eye, ocular inflammation, retinoblastoma, and malignant tumors of the anterior segment are contraindications to keratoplasty.

The European Eye Bank Association (EEBA) has set medical standards (table 1 and 2) which are reviewed every year. They can be considered as the minimum to be checked before considering a deceased patient as a potential donor of ocular tissue. They are available at the website of the association (www.europeaneyebanks.org). Other scientific societies such as the Eye Bank Association of America and the Eye Bank Association of Australia and New Zealand have set their own medical standards which are not significantly different from the European standards.

Table 1. EEBA medical standards

Information required for donor risk assessment
Donor's identity and age
Cause, time and circumstances of death
Past and recent medical history
Behavioral activity that increases the risk of transmissible diseases
Sources of information
Medical records
Attending medical and nursing staff
Family members or other relevant persons close to the deceased
Family doctor
Physical examination of the donor
Postmortem report if available and timely (when autopsy is performed)
Microbiological testing of donors
As a minimum, seronegativity for the following tests is required
HIV-1 and -2 antibody
Hepatitis B surface antigen
Hepatitis C virus antibody
Syphilis
Tests should be performed on a blood sample collected as soon as possible after death; the sample should be examined for hemolysis; if the donor has received infusions within the last 48 h, the volumes must be recorded and an algorithm applied to assess hemodilution; alternatively, an antemortem blood sample taken before any transfusions or infusions, and up to 7 days before the donation, may be available for testing
Heavy immunosuppression may invalidate serological antibody tests
Donor age and postmortem time
Provided that corneas are examined to exclude those with inadequate endothelium, no upper donor age limit needs to be set, but other age-related corneal changes must be taken into account; the lower age limit is less certain and will depend on surgical demand
It is recommended that corneal preservation occurs as soon as possible after death; all time intervals for each donor (death to enucleation and preservation) shall be recorded

The European Eye Bank Association Medical Standards

These medical standards include the information required for donor risk assessment, the relevant sources of information, microbiological testing of donors and contraindications to ocular tissue transplantation. No upper limit is set for donor age in these standards (table 1). Many clinical studies showed that donor age has no influence on graft survival [1–6]. In one study organ-cultured corneas from older donors were associated with higher graft survival [7]. The corneal endothelium in elderly donors has been shown to be more stable during organ culture [8] which could imply higher resistance to postoperative endothelial stress. Conversely, donor age influences the

Table 2. EEBA medical standards: contraindications to ocular tissue transplantation

Infections
AIDS/HIV
Active viral hepatitis (A, B, C)
Seropositivity: HIV, hepatitis B surface antigen, hepatitis C virus, syphilis
Behavior leading to risk of contracting HIV, hepatitis B or C
Having sex with someone who has (or thinks they have) AIDS or who is HIV positive
Men having sex with another man
Working as a prostitute
Injecting drugs, even once
Within the last 12 months: having sex with someone who has participated in the above high-risk activities; having sex with someone, of any race, living in Africa (except Morocco, Algeria, Tunisia, Libya or Egypt); tattooing, acupuncture, ear or body piercing; imprisonment
Viral encephalitis or encephalitis of unknown origin, viral meningitis
Rabies
Congenital rubella
Reye's syndrome
Tuberculosis (active disease or within first 6 months of treatment)
Progressive multifocal leukoencephalopathy
Septicemias: viremia and viral meningitis are absolute contraindications; bacterial forms of septicemia or meningitis may be acceptable at the discretion of the eye bank medical director but only when the corneas are to be stored by organ culture; additional microbiological testing is required
Jaundice of unknown etiology
HTLV-1 and -2 infection
Active malaria
Receipt of an organ transplant
Unknown etiology and CNS disorders
Creutzfeldt-Jakob disease and the following risk groups
Family history
Recipients of dura mater or brain/spinal surgery before August 1992
Recipients of human pituitary-derived hormones
CNS diseases of unknown etiology (e.g. multiple sclerosis, Alzheimer's disease, other dementias)
Subacute sclerosing panencephalitis (slow infection caused by measles virus with symptoms resembling Creutzfeldt-Jakob disease)
Chronic fatigue syndrome
Death from unknown cause is not a contraindication provided a postmortem examination is pending, and the result will be known before the tissue is transplanted
Malignancies and premalignancies
Leukemia
Lymphoma
Myeloma

Table 2. Continued

Eye disease and ocular surgery
Ocular inflammation (including known ocular involvement by systemic disease, e.g. sarcoidosis, rheumatoid arthritis)
Congenital or acquired disorders of the eye or previous ocular surgery (including corneal laser surgery) that would prejudice graft outcome
Retinoblastoma
Malignant tumors of the anterior segment
Receipt of a corneal, scleral or limbal graft
Scleral and limbal tissues
Use of preserved scleral tissue: donor medical assessment is the same as for corneas
Use of limbal tissues for keratolimbal allografts: donor medical assessment is the same as for corneas; malignancies represent additional contraindications because the limbus is vascularized

percentage of donor tissue discarded for endothelial reasons during storage. The higher the donor age, the lower the percentage of corneas accepted for penetrating keratoplasty.

Rationale for Contraindications to Ocular Tissue Transplantation

Viral and Prion Infections

Contraindications to ocular tissue transplantation include neurological diseases which may be transmissible to the recipient and those with unclear pathophysiology: rabies, contact with rabies virus, spongiform encephalitis (sporadic, inherited and iatrogenic Creutzfeldt-Jakob disease, CJD; Gerstmann-Stäussler-Scheinker syndrome; kuru), family history of spongiform encephalitis, recipients of human pituitary-derived hormones before 1987, surgery using dura mater, brain/spinal surgery before August 1992, CNS diseases of unknown etiology (e.g. multiple sclerosis, Alzheimer's disease, other dementias, Guillain-Barré syndrome), progressive multifocal leukoencephalopathy, amyotrophic lateral sclerosis, Reye's syndrome, congenital rubella, subacute sclerosing panencephalitis, viral encephalitis or encephalitis of unknown origin, viral meningitis.

Donor-to-host transmission of rabies and CJD is well established, and it is lethal for the recipient. Eight cases of recipient death after transplantation of donor tissue contaminated with the rabies virus have been reported [9–12]. For CJD, 1 reported case of recipient death is likely due to donor-to-recipient transmission of prions, and 2 further cases may correspond to transmission of prions [13–15]. In the first case the donor cause of death was CJD, and CJD occurred in the recipient who died 27 months after transplantation. In the further 2 cases, the recipient presented CJD and died but in 1 case no information concerning the donor was available and in the other case the delay between surgery and recipient death was quite long (i.e. 30 years). Clinically, these cases featured no major memory loss, disorders of higher cerebral functions or extrapyramidal signs, while cerebellar abnormalities were more frequent. Progressive dysarthria and gait disorder/gait ataxia were prominent signs during the early stages, myocloni the most salient feature later [16]. The risk of a prion-infected corneal donor appearing in the donor pool in the USA was shown to be 2 cases/year (0.005% of all donors) [17]. If donors with a characteristic quadrate clinical prodrome including cognitive changes, speech abnormalities, cerebellar findings and myoclonus and any patient undergoing autopsy for evaluation of possible CNS disease are to be excluded, the risk of inclusion of CJD-infected transplant tissues derived from ocular sources is very small, and all previously reported cases would have been prospectively excluded from surgical use.

Currently no biological detection of rabies virus and prions is routinely performed before delivering human donor corneal tissue for transplantation. Only clinical donor selection can discard donors at risk of transmitting these infectious agents. It seems logical to discard not only donors with one of these diseases (clinically evident or latent), but also those with symptoms which may resemble rabies or CJD.

It has been established that hepatitis B virus can be transmitted by corneal transplantation. Two cases of postoperative hepatitis B in the recipient starting respectively 2 and 4 months after surgery have been reported after transplantation of corneas from hepatitis-B-surface-antigen-positive donors [18]. Fortunately, no cases of recipient death have been reported after donor-to-recipient transmission of hepatitis B virus.

Donor-to-recipient transmission of herpes simplex virus is currently a major concern in terms of corneal transplantation safety [19]. It can induce primary graft failure, lack of graft reepithelialization, postoperative herpetic keratitis or postoperative keratouveitis [20–22]. However, in cases of postkeratoplasty herpetic infection, it is still difficult to ascertain whether the virus was transmitted in the donor tissue, reactivated in the recipient or infected the eye de novo after transplantation. Donor corneal tissue may contain the virus which was reported using the polymerase chain reaction to detect herpes simplex virus (HSV) thymidine kinase or HSV DNA in donor tissue [23, 24]. In fluid samples derived from 451 organ-cultured corneas, HSV-1 DNA corresponding to either the glycoprotein D or the thymidine kinase could be detected in 7 cases [25]. Currently no detection of HSV is routinely performed before delivering human donor corneal tissue for transplantation. Only donor selection can discard donors at risk of transmitting the virus. Several clinical reports strongly support the possible transmission of HSV via donor corneas. HSV-1 DNA was isolated in donor corneal buttons from 7 cases out of 21 primary graft failures, whereas HSV-2 DNA and varicella-zoster virus DNA were not found [21]. In 5 of these 7 cases, the recipient corneal tissue was negative for HSV-1 DNA, suggesting donor-to-host transmission of the virus. There are several reports of postkeratoplasty HSV infection in patients with no history of herpetic infection [19]. Lastly, transmission of HSV-1 by corneal transplantation has been demonstrated in a patient by means of genetic characterization of the virus [22]. As there is no biological test efficient to detect donor corneas with transmissible infectious HSV, only the clinical donor selection can currently discard dangerous donor tissue.

HIV infection, syphilis, hepatitis C, hepatitis A, tuberculosis (active disease or within first 6 months of treatment), HTLV-1 and -2 infection, active leprosy, active typhoid, smallpox and active malaria are contraindications to ocular tissue transplantation. However, no cases of transmission of one of these infectious agents via corneal grafts have been reported.

When organ culture is used for corneal storage, bacterial septicemias are not contraindications to corneal tissue transplantation. In fact, aqueous humor contamination is rare during bacterial septicemias, and organ culture permits detection of contaminated corneas before delivering tissue for transplantation [26]. Conversely, if hypothermic storage is to be used, bacterial septicemias have to be considered as contraindications to transplantation. Transmission of bacteria and fungi by corneal transplantation has been reported, and it may result in postoperative keratitis or endophthalmitis [27]. In clinical practice, the reported cases were grafts using donor corneal tissue stored at 4°C [28, 29]. The risk of bacteria or fungus donor-to-recipient transmission seems to be very low when organ culture is used for corneal storage. One isolated case of *Torulopsis glabrata* transmission via organ-cultured corneal grafting has been reported in 1978 in the USA [30]. No microbiological quarantine period was respected in this case, and no closed bottles were used for corneal storage. Current organ culture techniques make the risk of bacterial and fungal contamination of donor tissue very low.

Malignancies

Recipients of corneal tissue obtained from donors with malignancies do not have a higher risk of cancer than patients in the general population [31–33]. There is no evidence from reported clinical studies that recipients of corneal tissue obtained from eyes with choroidal melanoma have a higher risk of developing melanomas [31]. However, donor-to-recipient transmission of retinoblastoma has been reported. Retinoblastoma and malignant tumors of the anterior segment are contraindications to ocular tissue transplantation. Considering their high potential of dissemination [34, 35], leukemia, lymphoma and myeloma are considered as contraindications too.

Eye Disease and Ocular Surgery

Pseudophakic donor eyes with posterior chamber intraocular lenses have corneal endothelium qualities similar to phakic donor eyes, and they can be accepted for surgery [36]. Conversely, a history of corneal refractive surgery in a donor eye is a contraindication to keratoplasty. This is a difficult point as detecting corneal refractive surgery in donor corneas is not easy and needs further scientific developments. Other eye conditions which are contraindications to transplantation include ocular inflammation and receipt of a corneal, scleral or limbal graft.

The European Union Standards

The European Union directive on setting standards of quality and safety for donation, procurement, testing, processing, preservation, storage and distribution of human tissues and cells is the legal reference for donor selection in the European Union. The medical standards set in this directive (Commission Directive 2006/17/EC of February 8, 2006) are close to those of the EEBA. However, they include in addition:

- cause of death unknown, unless autopsy provides information on the cause of death after procurement;
- history of a disease of unknown etiology;
- systemic infection (viral, fungal or parasitic infections) which is not controlled at the time of donation;
- history of chronic, systemic autoimmune disease that could have a detrimental effect on the quality of the tissue to be retrieved;
- evidence of any other risk factors for transmissible diseases on the basis of a risk assessment, taking into consideration donor travel and exposure history and local infectious disease prevalence;
- presence on the donor's body of physical signs implying a risk of transmissible disease(s);
- ingestion of, or exposure to, a substance (such as cyanide, lead, mercury, gold) that may be transmitted to recipients in a dose that could endanger their health;
- recent history of vaccination with a live attenuated virus where a risk of transmission is considered to exist, and
- transplantation with xenografts.

Conclusion

Corneal transplantation safety is widely dependent on clinical donor selection. The medical standards set by the different international scientific societies and the European Union are similar, and they have to be respected for the purpose of providing patients with safe donor corneal tissue.

References

1 Borderie V, Baudrimont M, Bourcier T, Laroche L, Touzeau O: Les greffes en ophtalmologie. Paris, Elsevier, 2004.

2 Sugar A, Gal RL, Beck W, Ruedy KJ, Blanton CL, Feder RS, Hardten DR, Holland EJ, Lass JH, Mannis MJ, O'Keefe MB, Cornea Donor Study Group: Baseline donor characteristics in the Cornea Donor Study: baseline donor characteristics in the Cornea Donor Study. Cornea 2005;24:389–396.

3 Boisjoly HM, Tourigny R, Bazin R, Laughrea PA, Bubé I, Chamberland G, Bernier J, Roy R: Risk factors of corneal graft failure. Ophthalmology 1993; 100:1728–1735.

4 Gain P, Thuret G, Chiquet C, Rizzi P, Pugniet JL, Acquart S, Colpart JJ, Le Petit JC, Maugery J: Cornea procurement from very old donors: post organ culture cornea outcome and recipient graft outcome. Br J Ophthalmol 2002;86:404–411.

5 Volker-Dieben HJ, Kok-Van Alphen CC, Landsbergen Q, Persijn GG: Different influences on corneal graft survival in 539 transplants. Acta Ophthalmol 1982;60:190–202.

6 Williams KA, Roder DR, Esterman A, Muehlberg SM, Coster DJ: Factors predictive of corneal graft survival: report from the Australian Corneal Graft Registry. Ophthalmology 1992;99:403–414.

7 Borderie VM, Scheer S, Touzeau O, Vedie F, Carvajal-Gonzalez S, Laroche L: Donor corneal tissue selection before penetrating keratoplasty. Br J Ophthalmol 1998;82:382–388.

8 Armitage WJ, Easty DL: Factors influencing the suitability of organ-cultured corneas for transplantation. Invest Ophthalmol Vis Sci 1997;38:16–24.

9 Houff SA, Burton RC, Wilson RW, Henson TE, London WT, Baer GM, Anderson LJ, Winkler WG, Madden DL, Sever JL: Human-to-human transmission of rabies virus by corneal transplant. N Engl J Med 1979;300:603–604.

10 Anonymous: Human-to-human transmission of rabies via corneal transplant – Thailand. MMWR Morb Mortal Wkly Rep 1981;30:473–474.

11 Gode GR, Bhide NK: Two rabies deaths after corneal grafts from one donor. Lancet 1988;ii:791.

12 Javadi MA, Fayaz A, Mirdehghan SA, Ainollahi B: Transmission of rabies by corneal graft. Cornea 1996;15:431–433.

13 DeVoe AG. Complications of keratoplasty: Am J Ophthalmol 1975;79:907–912.

14 Hogan RN, Brown P, Heck E, Cavanagh HD: Risk of prion disease transmission from ocular donor tissue transplantation. Cornea 1999;18:2–11.

15 Heckmann JG, Lang CJ, Petruch F, Druschky A, Erb C, Brown P, Neundorfer B: Transmission of Creutzfeldt-Jakob disease via a corneal transplant. J Neurol Neurosurg Psychiatry 1997;63:388–390.

16 Lang CJ, Heckmann JG, Neundorfer B: Creutzfeldt-Jakob disease via dural and corneal transplants. J Neurol Sci 1998;160:128–139.

17 Hogan RN, Brown P, Heck E, Cavanagh HD: Risk of prion disease transmission from ocular donor tissue transplantation. Cornea 1999;18 2–11.

18 Hoft RH, Pflugfelder SC, Forster RK Ullman S, Polack FM, Schiff ER: Clinical evidence for hepatitis B transmission resulting from corneal transplantation. Cornea 1997;16:132–137.

19 Borderie VM, Meritet JF, Chaumeil C, Rozenberg F, Baudrimont M, Touzeau O, Bourcier T, Laroche L: Culture-proven herpetic keratitis after penetrating keratoplasty in patients with no previous history of herpes disease. Cornea 2004;23:118–124.

20 Biswas S, Suresh P, Bonshek RE, Corbitt G, Tullo AB, Ridgway AE: Graft failure in human donor corneas due to transmission of herpes simplex virus. Br J Ophthalmol 2000;84:701–705.

21 Cockerham GC, Bijwaard K, Sheng ZM, Hidayat AA, Font RL, McLean IW: Primary graft failure: a clinicopathologic and molecular analysis. Ophthalmology 2000;107:2083–2090.

22 Remeijer L, Maertzdorf J, Doornenbal P, Verjans GM, Osterhaus AD: Herpes simplex virus 1 transmission through corneal transplantation. Lancet 2001;357:442.

23 Biney EE, Orrett FA: Screening of human corneas for herpes simplex virus by tissue culture and polymerase chain reaction. Jpn J Med Sci Biol 1997;50: 151–160.

24 Neufeld MV, Steinemann TL, Merin LM, Stroop WG, Brown MF: Identification of a herpes simplex virus-induced dendrite in an eye-bank donor cornea. Cornea 1999;18:489–492.

25 Garweg JG, Boehnke M: Low rate shedding of HSV-1 DNA, but not of infectious virus from human donor corneae into culture media. J Med Virol 1997;52:320–325.

26 Borderie VM, Laroche L: Microbiologic study of organ-cultured donor corneas. Transplantation 1998;66:120–123.

27 Leibowitz HM, Moore TE: Keratoplasty; in Leibowitz HM, Waring GO III (eds): Corneal Disorders: Clinical Diagnosis and Management. Philadelphia, Saunders, 1998, pp 842–869.

28 Kloess PM, Stulting RD, Waring GO, Wilson LA: Bacterial and fungal endophthalmitis after penetrating keratoplasty. Am J Ophthalmol 1993;115:309–316.

29 Sutphin JE, Pfaller MA, Hollis RJ, Wagoner MD: Donor-to-host transmission of *Candida albicans* after corneal transplantation. Am J Ophthalmol 2002;134:120–121.

30 Larsen PA, Lindstrom RL, Doughman DJ: *Torulopsis glabrata* endophthalmitis after keratoplasty with an organ cultured cornea. Arch Ophthalmol 1978;96:1019–1022.

31 Harrison DA, Hodge DO, Bourne WM: Outcome of corneal grafting with donor tissue from eyes with primary choroidal melanomas: a retrospective cohort comparison. Arch Ophthalmol 1995;113:753–756.

32 Salame N, Viel JF, Arveux P, Delbosc B: Cancer transmission through corneal transplantation. Cornea 2001;20:680–682.

33 Wagoner MD, Dohlman CH, Albert DM, Lavin P, Murphy A, O'Neill-Dryja M: Corneal donor material selection. Ophthalmology 1981;88:139–145.

34 McGeorge AJ, Vote BJ, Elliot DA, Polkinghorne PJ: Papillary adenocarcinoma of the iris transmitted by corneal transplantation. Arch Ophthalmol 2002;120:1379–1383.

35 Lopez-Navidad A, Soler N, Caballero F, Lerma E, Gris O: Corneal transplantations from donors with cancer. Transplantation 2007;83:1345–1350.

36 Meier FM, Tschanz SA, Ganzfried R, Epstein D: A comparative assessment of endothelium from pseudophakic and phakic donor corneas stored in organ culture. Br J Ophthalmol 2002;86:400–403.

Vincent M. Borderie, MD, PhD
Centre Hospitalier National d'Ophtalmologie des XV–XX
28, rue de Charenton
FR–75012 Paris (France)
Tel. +33 1 40021507, Fax +33 1 40021599, E-Mail borderie@quinze-vingts.fr

Bredehorn-Mayr T, Duncker GIW, Armitage WJ (eds): Eye Banking.
Dev Ophthalmol. Basel, Karger, 2009, vol 43, pp 31–46

Organ Culture Preservation for Corneal Tissue

Technical and Quality Aspects

E. Pels · W.J. Rijneveld

Cornea Bank Amsterdam, Euro Tissue Bank, Amsterdam, The Netherlands

Abstract

Introduction: The technical and quality aspects of organ culture as a storage method for human donor corneas are described. **Materials and Methods:** Data electronically stored since 1989 of >41,000 corneas, processed in the Cornea Bank Amsterdam, are analysed. The technical information of eye banks collected in the Directory of the European Eye Bank Association (EEBA) is used as comparison. European Union (EU) directive for tissue banking and EEBA technical guidelines are references for the quality aspects. **Results:** Organ culture allows the storage of donor corneas up to 4–5 weeks. The storage phase is followed by a generally much shorter phase of 1–7 days, to reverse the corneal swelling occurring in the first phase and to transport the tissue to the clinic. Selection of the corneas based on inspection of the endothelium after storage as well as microbiological testing of the storage solution after a quarantine period are mandatory for this technique. General agreement exists about the outline of the method, but technical variations are applied to suit local circumstances and preferences of corneal surgeons. Agreement exists about a minimum endothelial cell count as selection criterion in case the donor endothelium is meant to be grafted. The use and cut-off points of other selection parameters for the cornea, e.g. the endothelial cell mosaic, are varying. According to EU regulations, a quality management system should be installed. This way each bank is able to issue a standardized product, while the production process is monitored with quality registrations. With the clinical outcome of the graft, the quality of the selection and storage procedures is verified. With the notification of adverse reactions such as primary graft failure and endophthalmitis, minimum risks will be assessed. **Conclusion:** The organ-cultured cornea is a well-documented product concerning microbiological safety and quality of the tissue. However, variations in performance and materials and no definite cut-off points for selection do not make an organ-cultured cornea a generally standardized product. The corneal surgeons have to ascertain themselves of the safety and quality of the followed procedure. It is up to an organization such as the EEBA to formulate tissue-specific additions to the EU regulations such as training opportunities, technical guidelines and criteria based on science.

Technical Aspects

General

Summerlin was the first to store a cornea by organ culture in 1973. Doughman et al. [1] however adapted it for eye banking to allow a storage time for corneas of 4–5 weeks before grafting. In his turn, Sperling [2] modified the technique of Doughman et al. and introduced organ culture in Europe in 1978. He added dextran T500 to the original storage solution. This addition prevented the corneal swelling in vitro and facilitated a closed system with microbiological testing of the storage medium before grafting. Sperling supposed that the high molecular weight of this dextran, 10 times higher than the dextran used in the media for cold storage, prevented its uptake by the cornea and the corneal cells. Grafting results were good; nevertheless, electron microscopy revealed that this dextran was also taken up and ingested by all corneal cells [3]. Another modification followed, and from that time onwards until today organ culture consists of two successive phases: storage in Doughman's medium, the longest phase, and a subsequent much shorter phase to reverse swelling in Sperling's medium, which is also used for transport at room temperature [4].

Sperling's other contribution to the storage of donor corneas by organ culture, the evaluation of the endothelium by light microscopy after swelling of the intercellular space, became inherent to this storage technique [5]. In addition to the medium-term storage period, it provides the advantage of delivering corneal tissue with a defined endothelial quality determined after storage.

Also a quarantine period to allow microbiological testing of the storage solution is inherent to the organ culture procedure. In this way, the vulnerability of organ cultures for microbes was exploited – microbiological contamination will be more readily evident – to reduce the risk of grafting contaminated corneal tissue [6].

Technical details, like storage temperature, composition of the basal medium, concentration of serum and dextran, antibiotics used, medium change and maximum storage period, differ between eye banks applying organ culture in Europe (Directory European Eye Bank Association, EEBA). The documented results and experiences demonstrate the common denominator of organ culture and the variations possible to adapt the technique to local circumstances and preferences of the involved corneal surgeons.

The organ culture storage technique performed by the Cornea Bank Amsterdam (CBA) is described below as an example to show the outline with the relatively uniform steps of the procedure. The performance of the steps aiming at the same result may differ however between banks, and references are made to these other methods.

Decontamination

Aim: Reduction of contaminating microbes from the donor cornea.

Retrieval of the donor tissue may occur by removal of the corneoscleral button in situ or by enucleation of the globe. In case of retrieval of globes, the bulbi are decontaminated on arrival in the bank.

With a running solution (fig. 1a), the number of microbes is significantly reduced. In the past, in the old location, tap water was used by the CBA. Since 1999, when the microbiological quality of the tap water turned out to be no longer standard and became a risk, it has been replaced by a sterile saline solution.

Tap water is still used by some banks, while others prefer sterile solutions.

A further reduction of the contaminating microbes is obtained by immersion in 0.5% polyvinylpyrrolidone-iodine solution for 2 min, followed by rinsing steps for 1 min in 0.5% thiosulphate solution and finally buffered saline. There are banks that prefer only the first or only the final step or the use of antibiotics in addition to the polyvinylpyrrolidone-iodine. The polyvinylpyrrolidone-iodine concentration may vary from 0.5 to 5%.

In case of removal of a corneoscleral button in situ, comparable variations in decontamination regimens are applied before the excision.

In both situations the decontamination is continued with the antibiotics in the storage solution.

A combination of penicillin, streptomycin and nystatin is preferred by the CBA for various reasons. The loss of corneas due to a contamination is <2%. This is considered acceptable by the CBA. Further reduction with more stable and wide-spectrum antibiotics has been balanced against the possible induction of multi-resistant microbes in an organ culture environment. Also it is considered as an advantage that stronger antibiotics are available in the clinic in case a contamination has passed undetected.

Most other banks use penicillin as well as streptomycin but amphotericin B instead of nystatin. A few banks prefer another class of antibiotics.

Evaluation of the Tissue

Aim: Selection of the tissue according to tissue-specific criteria to prevent graft failure. At first the cornea is macroscopically examined for clarity, epithelial integrity, foreign objects, opacities and colour of the sclera (such as jaundice). This is followed by slit-lamp examination (fig. 2a). The status concerning the presence of an arcus lipoides and the diameter of the clear zone, damage or erosions of the epithelium, scar(s) and stromal opacities with size, depth and their location in or out of the optic centre, number and depth of Descemet's folds, snail tracks and striae, signs of previous operations of the anterior segment such as cataract extraction, glaucoma surgery, refractive surgery, signs of pathology, e.g. cornea guttata, or inflammation are recorded.

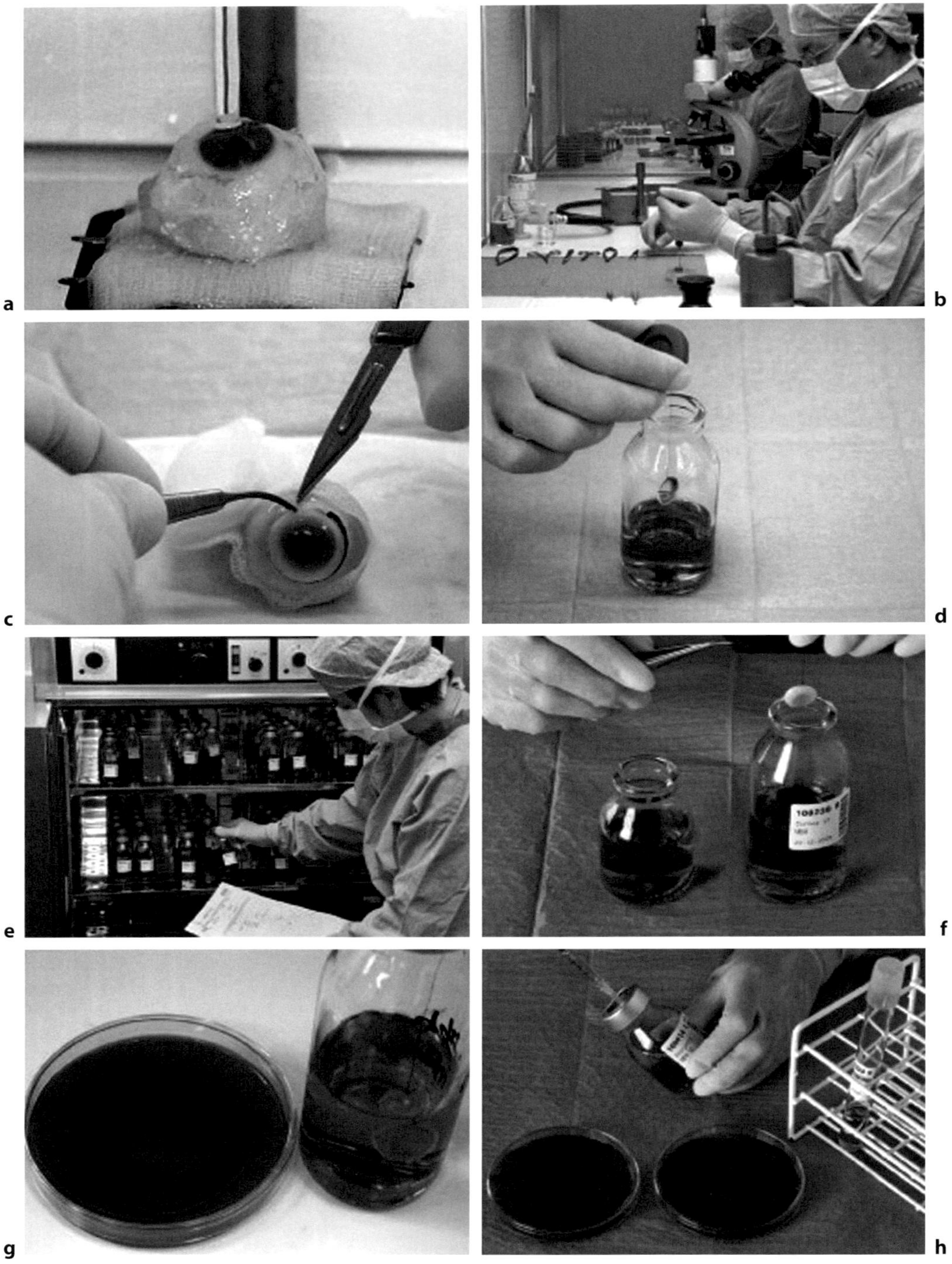
a
b
c
d
e
f
g
h

Following excision of the corneoscleral button (fig. 1c), the endothelium is inspected by light microscopy after staining with trypan blue and swelling of the intercellular space with a hypotonic solution at a magnification of ×125 (fig. 2b) [see chapter on the evaluation of the donor corneal endothelium for corneal organ culture by Schroeter and Rieck, this vol., pp. 47–62]. The whole surface of the endothelium is inspected, and relevant images are made. Cell density is estimated with the help of a graticule in one of the oculars and a nomogram. This is a graph where the cell density, assessed on images by manual counting according to Gundersen's method, is plotted against the number of cells determined on the lines of the graticule. Findings are recorded, such as the swelling pattern on and outside Descemet's folds, the presence of dead cells with nuclei stained by trypan blue, degenerating cells with granules in the cells, the distribution of these dead and dying cells indicative of intrinsic (postmortem damage) or extrinsic (enucleation, transport and excision) damage (fig. 2g, h) and the cell mosaic (fig. 2d). The status of the epithelium and keratocytes is also described. Mean corneal thickness of 5 spots in the centre is estimated by use of the micrometre screw of the microscope. The difference between the micrometre readings when first the epithelial side of the corneas is focused and then the endothelial side is correlated with the thickness of the cornea.

Before reversal of the corneal swelling by transferring the cornea to the transport medium, the evaluation of the endothelium by light microscopy is repeated. Special attention is paid to the condition of the endothelium on the preservation folds, the loss of cells during storage and the presence of reformation patterns indicative of cell loss [7]. Inspection of the endothelium after reversal of the swelling is not preferred by the CBA. The advantage of a cornea with fewer folds and a flatter surface that requires less focusing has been balanced against an additional handling of the cornea and extra recovery time before the transport after the induced intercellular swelling.

Other methods are used to visualize the endothelium. Trypan blue is not always used. Dead and degenerating cells can also be recognized without staining of the nuclei. But because trypan blue also stains the denuded Descemet's membrane, it helps to discriminate between areas without endothelium and areas where the endothelium is present but not visible because the intercellular space does not swell.

Different solutions are applied to visualize the endothelium by provoked swelling of the intercellular space. The pattern of this intercellular swelling may vary but each bank is accustomed to its own images. Staining of the cell membranes with alizarin red on a regular basis in experimental circumstances (fig. 2e, f) may be a great help

Fig. 1. Storage by organ culture. **a** Decontamination of the globe by rinsing. **b** Handling in the laminar airflow cabinet using aseptic techniques. **c** Excision of the corneoscleral button. **d** Corneoscleral button hanging in the culture medium by a suture attached to the stopper. **e** Storage in the incubator at 31°C (first phase). **f** Transfer of the corneoscleral button from the storage medium to the transport medium. **g** A blood agar plate showing growth of microbes in a sample of the medium while the storage medium concerned is still clear. **h** Sampling of the transport solution for microbiological testing.

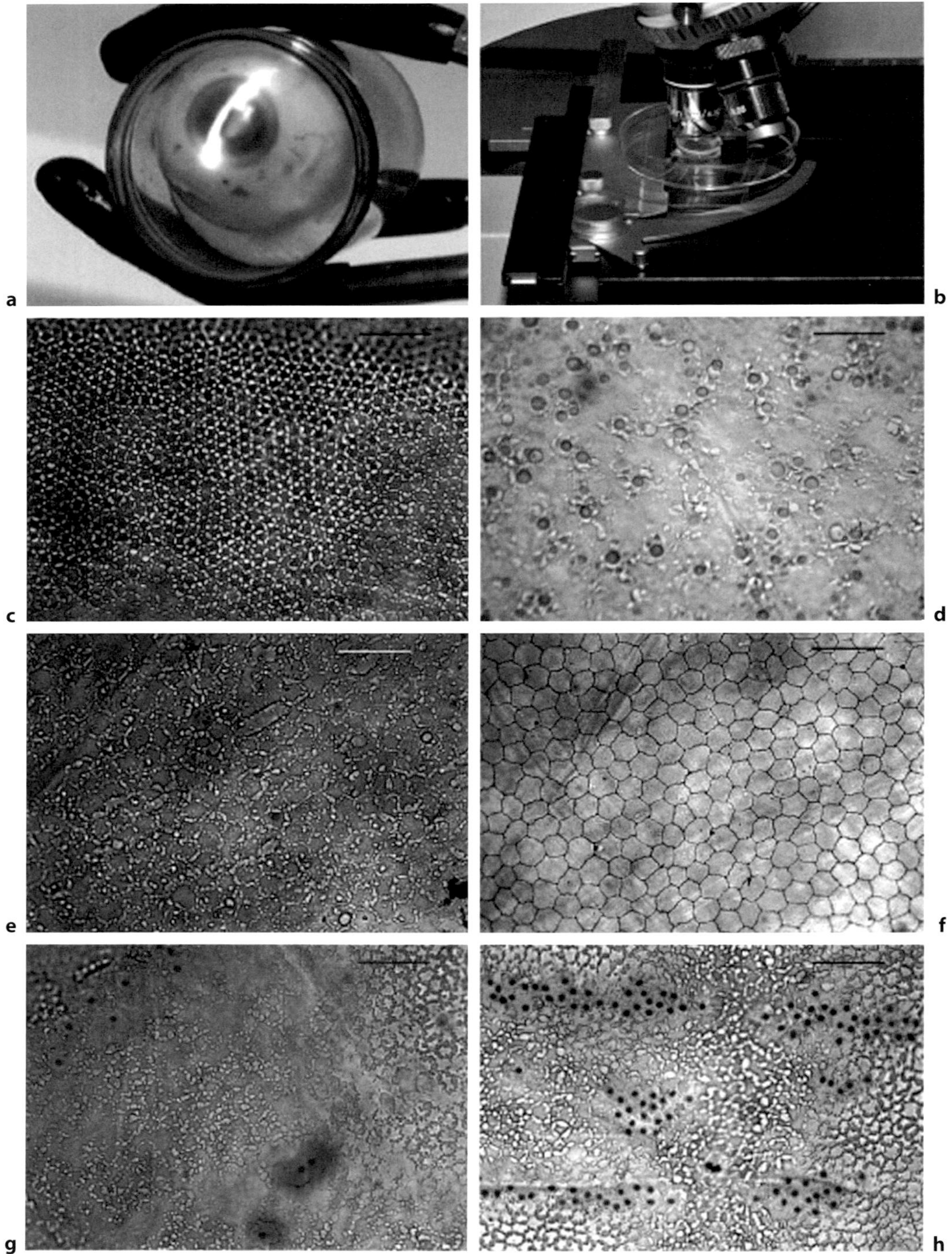

for the interpretation of the images and the training of the staff. The CBA prefers to include slit-lamp examination to inspect the general condition of the anterior segment of the donor eye. Inspection of the cornea with reflected light in addition to microscopic evaluation with transmitted light may be helpful, in particular to detect stromal opacities.

There are also banks that solely rely on microscopic evaluation after the first storage phase. Some prefer to inspect the endothelium after the reversal of the swelling.

In accordance with the EEBA Technical Guidelines, the condition of the epithelium, the stroma and the endothelium is checked. The vitality of the endothelium has been proven to be essential for graft transparency. Selection parameters are dependent on the surgical procedure for the intended kind of grafting: anterior or posterior lamellar; penetrating, either scheduled or emergency procedure; endothelium or Descemet's membrane. In the case of the CBA, definite cut-off points are agreed on with the Dutch corneal surgeons. Criteria for the endothelium are: >2,300 cells/mm^2, no or minimal polymegathism or pleiomorphism, cell loss <20% at the end of the first-phase storage period and normal cell morphology.

General agreement exists about the use of morphometric parameters of the endothelium for selection. As the specific influence of them on graft outcome remains uncertain, cut-off points are however at the discretion of the director. As a result the cut-off points may vary between banks, e.g. for cell count from 2,000 to 2,500 (EEBA Directory).

Storage

Aim: Maintenance of corneal viability, in particular of the endothelium, for a medium-term period of up to 4–5 weeks.

This storage period allows sufficient time for the performance of microbiological testing for safety, tissue typing and matching, recovery of reversible post-mortem damage and scheduling of the transplantation.

Fig. 2. Evaluation of the corneal tissue. **a** Slit-lamp examination of a cornea with an advanced arcus lipoides. **b** Examination of the corneal endothelium by light microscopy. Objective ×10, oculars ×12.5. **c–h** Images of the corneal endothelium. Scale bars = 0.1 mm. **c–e**, **g**, **h** After staining with trypan blue and artificial swelling of the intercellular space. **f** After staining of the intercellular borders with alizarin red. **c** Male, 24 years, 3,260 cells/mm^2, absence of polymegathism and pleiomorphism. **d** Female, 79 years, about 1,818 cells/mm^2, swelling of the intercellular space is incomplete, protrusions of Descemet's membrane, cornea guttata, stained with trypan blue. **e**, **f** Male, 68 years, 1,003 cells/mm^2 after cataract extraction and placement of an anterior chamber lens. **g** Female, 29 years, 3,072 cells/mm^2, cells with stained nuclei and stained denuded areas of Descemet's membrane. **h** Female, 59 years, 2,727 cells/mm^2, stained nuclei lying in rows indicating extrinsic damage due to folding; note the absence of the intercellular swelling in the neighbourhood of the stained cells.

Under aseptic conditions (fig. 1b) with the help of a trephine of 15–16 mm as preferred by the CBA, scissors, forceps and knife, the corneoscleral button is carefully excised (fig. 1c). After evaluation of the endothelium, the cornea is suspended in 50 ml culture medium by a suture attached to the inside of the impermeable stopper of a 100-ml glass vial (fig. 1d). It is stored in an incubator at 31°C for minimally 6 (quarantine period) and maximally 28–35 days (fig. 1e).

During storage, the cornea swells to about twice its normal thickness in 6–10 days. The swelling is more pronounced in tissue derived from younger donors [4].

In general the survival of the endothelium and the keratocytes is not affected, although exceptions may occur. Organ culture is considered as a stress test, and tissue with irreversibly affected vitality reveals itself by significant endothelial cell loss and necrosis of cells. The epithelial layer renews itself but is reduced to 2–3 cell layers. The superficial layers are shed off and are found as cellular debris at the bottom of the glass vial. This is the reason why the cornea is suspended in the medium and is not lying at the bottom.

Because the storage medium contains a pH indicator and the pH of the medium changes from 7.4 to 7.0 during storage, the colour of the medium changes from red orange to yellow orange.

Some banks prefer permeable stoppers or plastic vials and use a CO_2 incubator to maintain the pH. The nourishing conditions for the cornea are improved by renewal of the medium and larger volumes of medium.

With the increasing interest in lamellar grafting, the optimal storage conditions may be different dependent on the requirements: optimal survival of keratocytes, epithelium or endothelium. Storage conditions may also have to be adapted for corneoscleral buttons provided with a section plane by the bank, hand made, made with a microkeratome or intralase.

Reversal of the Swelling and Transport

Aim: Delivery of tissue that is sufficiently clear for surgical handling and regains its function as soon as possible after grafting.

Minimally 3 and maximally 7 days before surgery and after inspection of the endothelium, the cornea is transferred to the transport medium containing 5% dextran T500 (fig. 1f).

Reversal of the swelling is complete within 12–24 h. The time needed for the reversal is independent of the dextran concentration whereas the final thickness is determined by it. The handling of the cornea during inspection and transfer may restimulate the growth of remaining microbes. A quarantine period for another microbiological test at the expense of some accumulation of dextran in the cornea and the corneal cells has to be balanced against a short time between transfer and grafting to prevent these microbes to become a risk by growing. The preference is affected by the expected time of transport and the distribution area of a bank.

Transport occurs at room temperature. The dextran in the medium protects the endothelium from damage due to the lower than physiological temperature and fast movements of the cornea due to its viscosity.

The toxicity of dextran for the endothelium and the corneal cells is judged differently by banks. Whether this is caused by the source of the dextran, its purity and by-products, is not known. It has however consequences for the limits set for the transport phase. They vary from 1 to 7 days. Studies are performed for alternatives such as hydroxyethyl starch and poloxamers. The CBA considers the adherence of cellular debris from the epithelium to the endothelium a larger risk than the uptake and possible toxicity of the dextran and accepts 7 days in transport medium as a maximum. Whether the dextran might interfere with the adhering capacity of posterior corneal lamellae is however currently studied. Therefore the time period in dextran-containing medium is currently limited to 3 days in those cases.

Microbiological Testing of the Storage Solutions

Aim: Reduction of the risk of grafting a contaminated cornea, which might cause an adverse reaction in the graft of increasing severity, infection of the anterior segment, ocular infection and endophthalmitis.

Despite all decontamination procedures, contaminating microbes remain. Some will reveal themselves by a change in colour or clarity of the medium, while others might be present without a sign (fig. 1g).

A sample of the medium is taken after 3 days of storage. It is expected that the antibiotics should have done their job before they get instable and inactive. The medium sample is cultured for 7 days on blood agar plates at 35°C and room temperature and in tryptic soy broth at 35°C. This time period turned out to be too short to be fully safe; not all (about 84%) of the contaminants are detected. Therefore an additional test is performed on the day of transfer, after minimally 6 days of storage. The CBA tests the transport medium again 1 day after transfer of the cornea (fig. 1h). The handling of the storage medium and the cornea as well as the transfer to a new medium might stimulate remaining, still undetected microbes. As the transport time may increase up to 7 days, these microbes are a possible risk. Other banks prefer to reduce this time period to 1–2 days with the toxicity of the dextran as reason but also to reduce the microbiological risk that way. All test results should be negative on the day of shipment and the day of grafting (minimally 2 and 3 days after transfer, respectively).

The frequency of delivering a contaminated graft that needs additional treatment in the clinic has been less than 0.023%. One out of 22,019 grafts lost transparency.

The time schedule for the microbiological testing of the CBA is historically grown. Tests were added in the past whenever the test system needed improvements (1993 and 1999).

Other banks prefer other time schedules for sampling and other microbiological test methods, methods designed or adapted to their circumstances and conditions. In all cases a quarantine period that is documented to be safe and actual microbiological testing of the solutions are mandatory. Relying only on a change of colour and turbidity of the medium is not acceptable (fig. 1g).

Quality Aspects

General

Banks originated as supporting units to facilitate grafting. They have been transferred to production units to comply with European Union (EU) legislation. Corneal tissue should be a documented safe and standardized product. Quality management systems are nowadays mandatory. This means e.g. that process steps are documented in standard operating procedures. They are monitored, measured and analysed with the help of quality registrations. The results may be incentives for improvement.

According to current legislation, each eye bank shall deliver a cornea for grafting in a standardized way. The technical details of the production process are however not standard for all banks (see above) but adapted to local preferences. Selection criteria are described (EEBA Minimum Technical Guidelines) but definitive cut-off points are not available as links with graft outcome are not clearly demonstrated. Because the scientific support for only one ideal procedure or specific selection criterion is lacking, the corneas delivered for grafting by different banks do not necessarily have a standardized quality and safety. Corneal surgeons should be aware of these differences when accepting tissue from other sources than usual. The most important aspects are discussed below.

Microbiological Safety

The screening of the donor tissue for transferable diseases will be described in another chapter. Other aspects of safety are discussed here.

On the one hand the microbiological safety is affected by decontamination and microbiological testing procedures in the bank. On the other hand additional measures may be taken in the clinic.

According to EU regulations, the air quality during the processing of the cornea is considered a key factor in tissue processing.

In the CBA the handling of the corneoscleral button using aseptic techniques is performed under aseptic conditions provided by a laminar airflow cabinet with an air quality comparable to good manufacturing practice (GMP) grade A. The background environment is grade C as is the case in many eye banks.

The CBA performs a check for aseptic handling once each week. A cornea discarded for grafting at the second evaluation with no contaminants found in the first-phase medium is transferred to an antibiotic-free medium. Medium samples for microbiological tests are collected after 1 week. In 2 of >590 corneas, growth has been observed indicating a risk of less than 0.34% of contaminating the cornea by handling.

Since 1995 the air quality of the environment has been assessed by particle counting (large, >0.5 μm, and small, <0.5 μm). The number of colony-forming units has been assessed since 2000. Settle plates have been used since 2003. No correlation is observed with the percentage contamination (fig. 3a, b).

The results demonstrate and document that the current environment of GMP class C quality does not affect the microbiological quality and safety of the cornea. In this way the environment chosen by the CBA achieves the quality as prescribed by the Commission Directive 2006/86/EC.

Other banks claiming to work in clean rooms with GMP class A critical areas and GMP class B background do not always have less contamination (Directory EEBA 2007). This shows that other factors play a larger role.

The post-mortem retrieved cornea is generally contaminated. The effectiveness of the decontamination procedure and the microbiological testing should therefore be documented.

The effectiveness of the used decontamination procedures has been studied [8]. In addition the percentage of contaminated corneas is plotted for the four quarters of the year (fig. 4). A significant effect of season was not observed. The gradual decrease in contaminated tissue might reflect the use of standard operating procedures by the banks since 1995 and the tissue retrieval organization since 1998. On 3 occasions, a deviation of the general pattern was observed:

In 1993 one specific contaminant, *Bacillus,* was prominent and the observed frequency increased dramatically. It turned out that some of the bottles with nystatin suspension while delivered as sterile were contaminated. This contamination did not change colour or clarity of the medium, so it would not have been detected without microbiological tests of the medium (fig. 1g).

Less significant in this graph because of the scale of the y-axis, but requiring attention at that time, is the contamination in the second quarter of 1999. It is increased compared to the previous time period. In addition the presence of slowly growing microbes was remarkable. Evaluation of the water system showed that the microbiological quality of the tap water was seriously affected by another kind of processing of the water destined for the laboratories. The tap water was replaced by sterile phosphate-buffered saline (see Technical Aspects).

In 2001 the increase in contamination consisted of different types of bacteria belonging to the flora on donor eyes. An increased transport time with insufficient cooling of the donor tissue turned out to be the cause.

Banks should collect this kind of information and make it available for corneal surgeons [9, 10]. In this way they can judge the microbiological safety. Additional

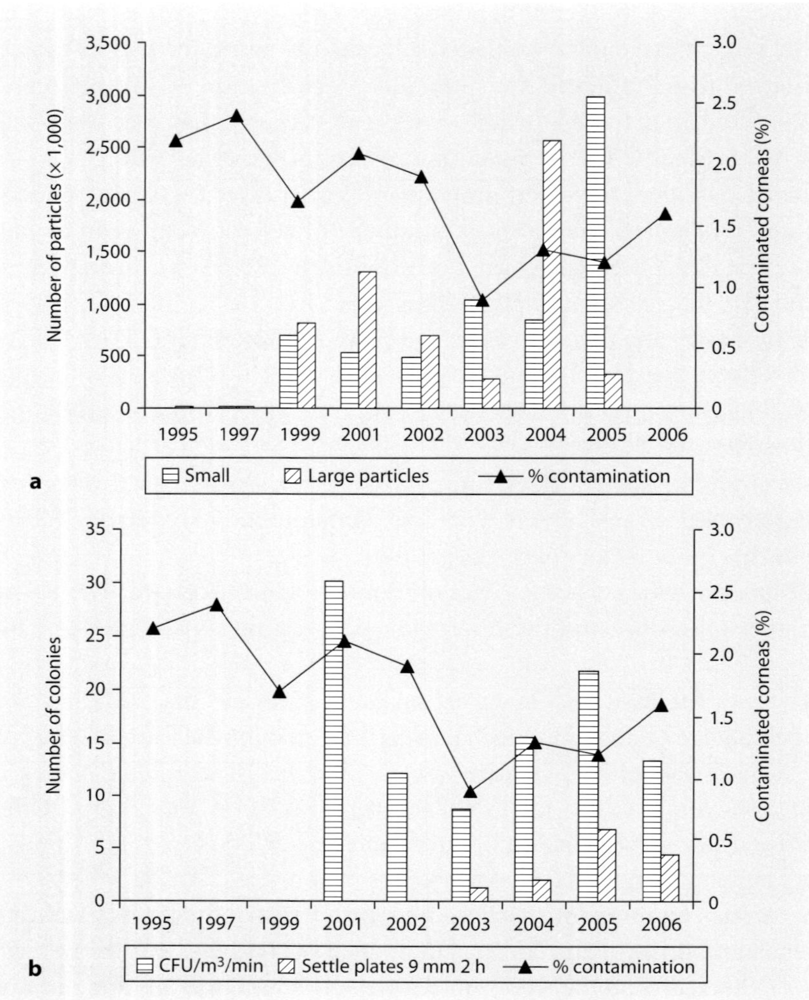

Fig. 3. Contamination of the cornea and the air quality of the process environment. The percentage of corneas detected as contaminated versus all stored corneas (right y-axis in the graphs) is plotted for consecutive years, in addition to the number of large and small particles per cubic foot per minute assessed in the air (**a**) and the number of colony-forming units (CFU) in the air with the number of colonies observed on settle plates (**b**).

measures may be considered, e.g. microbiological tests of the corneoscleral rim and transport medium, extended storage of the transport medium for tests later on when judged necessary, additional preventive antibiotic treatment.

By September 2007 Commission Directive 2006/86/EC shall be brought into force by the member states. This requires notification of serious adverse reactions to the competent authority. Grafting of a contaminated cornea resulting in affected graft

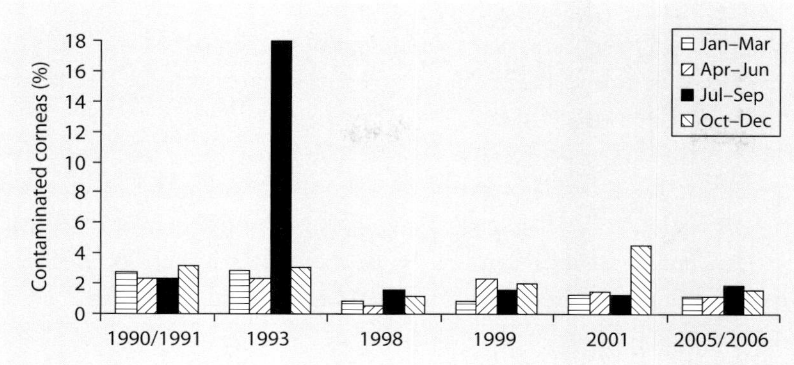

Fig. 4. Percentage of contaminated corneas over the years. The percentage of corneas detected as contaminated versus all stored corneas is plotted for the different quarters of the year.

outcome should be reported. Collection of this kind of information will show the actual risks.

Safety and Quality Affected by Storage Solutions

The storage solutions are critical materials and require documented specifications according to EU legislation (Commission Directive 2006/86/EC part C).

After the introduction of organ culture as a storage method, it took a long time before storage solutions became commercially available. In addition the used storage solutions differ in composition. Banks may therefore have a long history of producing these materials.

Since 1995 the CBA has produced its own storage solutions in a documented and well-controlled way. Produced batches are stored frozen until release and final use. Each batch consists of about 100 bottles with the fully composed storage solution, ready for use after thawing. Only the nystatin, being a suspension, has to be added. Before release each batch is extensively tested for microbiological safety. In addition the quality is tested with at least 5 human corneas not suitable for grafting. Experience has shown that minor changes in the composition or the origin of different basic substances may affect the vitality of the cornea. These modifications passed the quality control of the manufacturer unnoticed.

Since 1981 attention has been paid to the origin of the bovine serum to reduce the risk of prion disease. Serum batches have always been tested before use to exclude toxicity.

Considering standardization in general, commercially available products should be preferred. Agreement about the ideal composition does however not yet exist. So may the dextran concentration vary in the transport solutions (EEBA Directory). This affects the appearance of the corneal tissue, more or less swollen. It also affects the induction of the artificial swelling necessary to visualize the endothelium and by this the interpretation of the images. On the other hand, the production of storage solutions is not the core business of the manufacturers as it is for the eye banks that can test their products with the tissue itself.

In different centres media are developed and tested which are free of bovine serum. The development of these media is very important. From a safety point of view the risk of prion disease is reduced due to the replacement of the bovine products, provided the origin of the replacements is known. From a qualitative point of view, the replacement of the biological component serum by chemically better-defined products is an improvement.

Quality of Tissue Affected by Selection

For the transparency of the graft, a functioning endothelium is essential. A rationale has been presented for the setting of minimum donor cell densities by eye banks. This means that proper calibration of the microscope as well as evaluation of the counting results should be essential, irrespective of whether the counts are obtained manually or in a computer-assisted or fully automated manner [11, 12].

In the CBA the cell density is manually counted, and consistency is assessed at documented time intervals. The interobserver variation of 6 staff members is 3.2%. Lacking scientific support for other morphometric selection criteria, the evaluation of the endothelium should at least be standardized within the bank. Consistency in the judgement of the endothelial cell mosaic needs regular consultation between colleagues in the CBA. Documented training of staff is a key factor. Providing training courses might be a challenge for the EEBA.

Monitoring of the selection result, the percentage of corneas judged suitable for grafting versus the total number of donated corneas, has been another way in the CBA to test the consistency of selection (fig. 5). In 1998 the results have been improved by the introduction of a maximum age of 80 years for the donor because donor age has been shown to be an important factor [13, 14]. When in 2002 the selection result dropped, investigation showed that the vitality of the tissue was affected. After measures had been taken to improve tissue retrieval and transport, the selection result returned to the original level. A similar phenomenon has been described by another bank [15]. With the growing interest in lamellar grafting, it is expected that the results will change because tissue judged not suitable for a penetrating keratoplasty might be suitable for an anterior lamellar graft.

Utmost caution is warranted when selection results of individual banks per se are compared. They are dependent on many factors and preselections and are not indicative of the quality of tissue issued by a bank.

The final test for storage and selection is the clinical outcome. Clinical information about the corneas of patients grafted in the Netherlands has been collected and stored

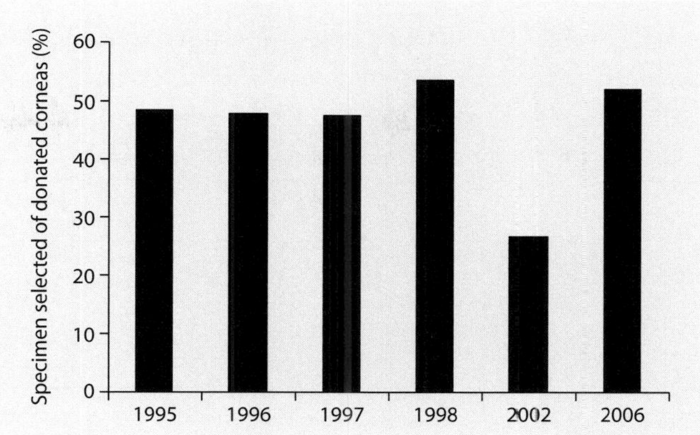

Fig. 5. Selection results. The percentage of selected corneas versus the donated corneas is plotted for a consecutive time period.

in a computer database since 1995. Of the 7,243 corneas transplanted up to July 2006, 4,424 have been followed minimally once (follow-up percentage 61%).

Eighteen corneas (0.41%) got cloudy within 1 month. Only 1 never cleared after grafting and is considered a primary graft failure. The others cleared first.

Other complaints are also collected as they may be a trigger for improvement.

For example, corneal surgeons started to complain about the presence of an arcus lipoides. A study of the graft size revealed that the arcus had not been overlooked in the bank but that the mean graft size in general was 7.5 mm. A clear diameter of less than 8 mm is nowadays judged as a contra-indication.

Banks in other countries do have their own follow-up registration (see EEBA Directory) and have published their results [16, 17]. In Australia [18] and Sweden, national graft registries are available collecting graft results of tissue processed by different banks.

The presence of such a register is an important tool for a bank in quality management. The storage and selection can be monitored. Results stimulate improvement.

According to EU legislation by 2008 all banks should have procedures in place to collect adverse reactions without delay. They have to notify nationally installed competent authorities of these events such as primary graft failure and endophthalmitis. Evaluation results should be reported as well. In this way a minimum level will be ensured.

Conclusion

The organ-cultured cornea is a well-documented product concerning microbiological safety and quality of the tissue. General agreement exists about the outline of the storage technique and selection parameters. However, variations in performance and materials, and the absence of definite cut-off points during selection, make the organ-cultured cornea not yet a fully standardized product.

Training of the staff by the EEBA may stimulate the standardization insofar as a living cornea may be considered a standard product.

References

1 Doughman DJ, Harris JE, Schmitt KM: Penetrating keratoplasty using 37°C organ-cultured cornea. Trans Am Acad Ophthalmol Otol 1976;81:778–793.

2 Sperling S: Human corneal endothelium in organ culture: the influence of temperature and medium of incubation: Acta Ophthalmol 1979;57:269–276.

3 Van der Want HJL, Pels E, Schuchard Y, Olesen B, Sperling S: Electron microscopy of cultured human corneas: osmotic hydration and the use of a dextran fraction (dextran T 500) in organ culture. Arch Ophthalmol 1983;101:1920–1926.

4 Pels E, Schuchard Y: Organ culture in the Netherlands: preservation and endothelial evaluation; in Brightbill FS (ed): Corneal Surgery: Theory, Technique and Tissue, ed 2. St Louis, Mosby Co, 1993, pp 622–632.

5 Sperling S: Assessment of endothelial cell density in bovine corneas after osmotically induced dilation of intercellular spaces. Cornea 1985/1986;4:71–79.

6 Armitage WJ, Easty DL: Factors influencing the suitability of organ-cultured corneas for transplantation. Invest Ophthalmol 1997;38:16–24.

7 Sperling S: Early morphological changes in organ cultured human corneal endothelium. Acta Ophthalmol 1978;56:785–792.

8 Pels E, Vrensen GFJM: Microbial decontamination of human donor eyes with povidone-iodine: penetration, toxicity, and effectiveness. Br J Ophthalmol 1999;83:1019–1026.

9 Borderie VM, Laroche L: Microbiologic study of organ-cultured donor corneas. Transplantation 1998;66:12–123.

10 Zanetti E, Bruni A, Mucignat G, Camposampiero D, Frigo AC, Ponzin D: Bacterial contamination of human organ-cultured corneas. Cornea 2005:24: 603–607.

11 Armitage WJ, Dick AD, Bourne WM: Predicting endothelial cell loss and long-term corneal graft survival. Invest Ophthalmol 2003;44:3326–3331.

12 Thuret G, Manissolle C, Acquart S, Le Petit J-C, Maugery J, Campos-Guyotat, Doughty MJ: Is manual counting of corneal endothelial cell density in eye banks still acceptable? The French Experience. Br J Ophthalmol 2003;87:1481–1486.

13 Armitage WJ, Easty DL: Factors influencing the suitability of organ-cultured corneas for transplantation. Invest Ophthalmol 1997;38:16–24.

14 Pels E, Beekhuis WH, Völker-Dieben HJ: Long term tissue storage for keratoplasty; in Brightbill FS (ed): Corneal Surgery: Theory, Technique and Tissue, ed 3. St Louis, Mosby Co, 1999, pp 897–906.

15 Ponzin D, Griffioni C, Fasolo A, Veronese A, Firgo C, Jones GLA: Eye banking at the Fondazione Banca degli Occhi Veneto: activities and perspectives. Organs Tissues 2003;2:11–19.

16 Vail A, Gore SM. Bradley BA, Easty DL, Rogers CA: Corneal graft survival and visual outcome: a multicenter study. Ophthalmology 1994;101:120–127.

17 Fasolo A, Frigo AC, Böhm E, Genisi C, Rama P, Spadea L, Mastropirro B, Fornea M, Ponzin D, Grigoletto F: The CORTES study: corneal transplant indications and graft survival in an Italian cohort of patients. Cornea 2006:25:507–515.

18 Williams KA, Muehlberg SM, Lewis RF, Coster DJ: Influence of advanced recipient and donor age on the outcome of corneal transplantation. Br J Ophthalmol 1997;81:835–839.

E. Pels, PhD
Cornea Bank Amsterdam, Euro Tissue Bank
p/a NIN Meibergdreef 47
NL–1105 BA Amsterdam (The Netherlands)
E-Mail e.pels@nin.knaw.nl

Bredehorn-Mayr T, Duncker GIW, Armitage WJ (eds): Eye Banking.
Dev Ophthalmol. Basel, Karger, 2009, vol 43, pp 47–62

Endothelial Evaluation in the Cornea Bank

Jan Schroeter · Peter Rieck

Cornea Bank Berlin, Clinic of Ophthalmology, Charité – Universitätsmedizin Berlin, Campus-Virchow-Klinikum, Berlin, Germany

Abstract

The light microscope is the first-choice technique for the evaluation of organ-cultured donor corneas. For the microscopic visualization of the endothelial cells, the corneas have to be immersed in a hypotonic solution. The number of cells, their vitality and morphology are analyzed. The cell density is easily estimated with the fixed frame/L method. Use of an image analysis system enables computer processing and counting of digitalized endothelial cell images. An adequately high endothelial cell density after the culture period is a decisive criterion that must be met before releasing a donor cornea for grafting. An endothelial cell density of 2,000–2,200 cells/mm^2 is generally recognized as the lower limit for the longest possible graft survival. While an evaluation of the endothelium does not necessarily have to be performed at the beginning or middle of organ culture, it is obligatory at the end. Morphology assessment should routinely involve estimating the pleomorphism (deviation from hexagonality), polymegathism (variation in cell area) and granulation/vacuolization of the endothelial cells. Recognition of devitalized cells is easily facilitated by vital staining with trypan blue.

Structure, Physiology and Function of the Corneal Endothelium

The endothelium is the metabolically most active as well as the most vulnerable layer of the human cornea. It consists of a single layer of cells (4–6 μm thick) that originates from the mesoderm. The endothelial cells are polygonal with 5–7 borders, mostly hexagonal. They have a diameter of about 22 μm and a surface area of about 250 μm^2. On their side facing the anterior chamber, they have 20–30 microvilli leading to a significant enlargement of the surface. The cell borders are connected via zonulae occludentes and adherentes and interdigitate and overlap. The endothelial cells have a flattened nucleus and all organelles for active transport and protein synthesis: rough and smooth endoplasmic reticulum, mitochondria and Golgi apparatus [1].

Immunocytochemical examinations have shown that the term 'endothelium' is actually misleading, since the cells possess none of the typical endothelial markers (no Weibel-Palade bodies, no factor VIII expression). The cytochemical pattern more closely resembles that of corneal epithelial cells (markedly positive labeling with antibodies against keratin, vimentin, S-100 protein and neuron-specific enolase) [2].

Endothelial cells show a marked physiological density decrease from the rim to the center of the cornea and an increase in pleomorphism [1, 3]. The central endothelial density decreases with age. Thus, it amounts to about 3,500–4,000 cells/mm^2 in newborns but only reaches levels of about 1,500–2,500 cells/mm^2 in older adults. However, advancing age is not the only cause of a marked endothelial cell loss; it can also result from eye operations, eye diseases and injuries. Human corneal endothelial cells are a postmitotic tissue with an extremely low proliferation rate. Thus, cell loss cannot be compensated by cell division but only by an increase in the size of the remaining adjacent endothelial cells. This inevitably leads to an irregular increase in the size of the endothelial cells and to a loss of the typical hexagonality. Progressive pleomorphism and polymegathism of endothelial cells are typical signs of an aged cornea.

Corneal transparency and thus the visual function of the eye are primarily ensured by the relative corneal dehydration, which is maintained by various mechanisms localized largely in the corneal endothelium. Nearly 130 years ago, Leber [4] already demonstrated that the endothelial cell layer prevents aqueous influx into the corneal stroma. We now have a more precise knowledge of the basic mechanisms. The two main endothelial cell functions are the maintenance of corneal dehydration by active, i.e. energy-dependent, pump mechanisms (Na^+-K^+-ATPase) and the physical barrier function ('leaky barrier') that characterizes fluid and electrolyte influx. The energy-dependent Na^+-K^+-ATPase removes fluid flowing into the stroma through the 'leaky' barrier.

A net influx could be demonstrated for Na^+ and HCO^{3-} but not for Cl^- or K^+ [5]. This ion flow establishes an osmotic gradient that causes water to flow from the stroma back into the aqueous. The pump mechanism is active, which means it is an energy-consuming metabolic process that can be inhibited by a temperature reduction. Other important endothelial functions are to synthesize Descemet's membrane and to supply the cornea with nutritive substances by diffusion of glucose, amino acids and other substances. The endothelial cells themselves are fed mainly by aqueous components but also by tear fluid.

Practical Implementation of Endothelial Assessment

Donor corneal endothelium is microscopically assessed. This is done with a light microscope, but a specular microscope is also suitable.

Light Microscopy

The light microscope is the first-choice technique for organ culture. An inverse microscope is particularly well suited for this purpose (e.g. CKX41, Olympus). The phase contrast technique is recommended, since it enables very high-contrast imaging of the unstained endothelial cell layer. A good combination is to use 100-fold magnification for a survey (visible endothelial area of about 1.2 mm^2) and 200-fold magnification for detailed images and cell counts (visible endothelial area of about 0.3 mm^2). Details are better visualized at 400-fold magnification, but the assessable area is very small. Low magnifications, e.g. 4-fold, enable imaging of the entire endothelial area; due to the natural corneal curvature, however, only a small part can be focused, and single cells are not recognizable.

For the microscopic examination, the cornea is placed in a sterile, closed and transparent vessel like a tissue culture dish (e.g. BD Falcon™ cell culture dish 35 × 10 mm) or tissue culture plate (e.g. BD Falcon 6-well cell culture plate) in medium or electrolyte solution covering fully the endothelial side of the cornea. Applying a closed system permits microscopy outside the laminar airflow. During microscopy, care must be taken to maintain sterile conditions inside the vessel. For microscopy with the inverse light microscope, the cornea is placed in the vessel with either the endothelium (the cornea is situated on the residual scleral rim) or the epithelium turned toward the lens. Positioning the donor cornea on the scleral rim enables better and more extensive imaging of the endothelial cell layer, since stromal compression folds are thus avoided. The working distance, i.e. the distance between the object and the lens, is important for corneal microscopy, since the cornea has a domed shape and is thus a certain distance away from the lens. This distance is also dependent on the width of the scleral rim. Since the working distance differs from microscope to microscope, not all types are equally well suited for use in the cornea bank. If the endothelial cells cannot be centrally focused (the point farthest away from the lens) when positioning the donor cornea on the scleral rim, it should be placed on the epithelial side. Which positioning enables better visualization is thus dependent on the microscope applied and can easily be determined by comparison. When procuring a microscope for the cornea bank, its suitability for that purpose must be confirmed beforehand.

A standard light microscope can also be used. Here the cornea must be placed on the epithelial side, since the lens of the microscope is over the cornea. This involves a very high risk of damaging the donor cornea or contaminating it with microorganisms, since the lens is situated directly over the unprotected endothelial cell layer because of the short working distance. This technique should therefore be avoided in the cornea bank and restricted to experimental studies.

Specular Microscopy

Endothelial microscopy can also be done with a specular microscope (e.g. Eye Bank Kerato Analyzer EKA-98, Konan Medical Inc.). This technique is used primarily for short-term culture (hypothermic storage). Specular microscopes semiautomatically

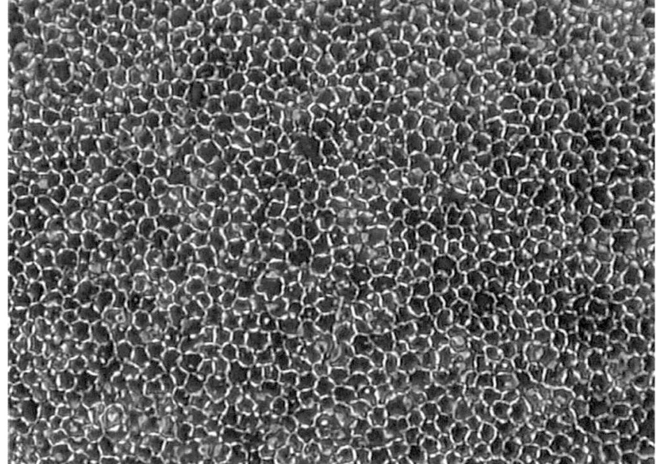

Fig. 1. Regular endothelium of a human donor cornea before organ culture. Hypotonic BSS, inverse microscope with phase contrast technique. Magnification ×200.

or automatically generate images of the endothelial cell layer after manually positioning the donor cornea. While virtually all areas of the donor cornea can be examined by light microscopy, this cannot be done with a specular microscope. Here the assessable area is usually restricted to the center of the cornea. Moreover, the visualized areas are relatively small because of a fixed apparatus-related magnification. In contrast to light microscopy however, specular microscopy does not require osmotic stimulation of the endothelial cells; thus, the donor cornea can remain in its storage vessel and culture medium (e.g. Optisol-containing vial, Chiron Ophthalmics).

To visualize endothelial cells by light microscopy, the cornea must be placed in osmotic solutions. Good results have been achieved here by using hypotonic BSS (balanced salt solution) with the following composition: 4.90 g of NaCl, 0.75 g of KCl, 0.49 g of $CaCl_2H_2O$, 0.30 g of $MgCl_26H_2O$, 3.90 g of sodium acetate $3H_2O$ and 1.70 g of sodium citrate $2H_2O$ dissolved in 1,000 ml of water for injection, pH approximately 7.76, osmolarity (osmolality) 0.25 osm/kg, conductance approximately 12.0 mS/cm. The cornea is placed under the microscope in a suitable vessel filled with sterile hypotonic BSS. After a few seconds, the cells swell, and their borders become clearly visible (fig. 1). The cornea should not be left in the hypotonic solution for longer than 5 min in order to minimize the risk of osmotic damage to the sensitive endothelium. Thus, the cornea should only be placed in the hypotonic solution right before microscopy and transferred to a suitable isotonic medium immediately after the examination. Assessment of several corneas should be done accordingly one after another.

An osmotic influence can also be exerted by 0.9 and 0.45% sodium chloride solution, Ringer's lactate solution and 1.8% sucrose solution (1.8 g of sucrose in 100 ml of water for injection, osmolality of 0.053 osm/kg). Any osmotic stress will irreversibly damage some endothelial cells and should thus be minimized. No negative influence on endothelial cell density was found for 0.45% sodium chloride solution and hypotonic BSS. In contrast a 1.8% sucrose solution reduced the endothelial cell density by a mean of 10% in the same time [6]. For routine diagnostics, it is advisable to select the solution that has the highest hypoosmolality but still enables good visualization of the endothelial cell layer and to keep the examination time at a minimum. An isotonic BSS mixed with 1.8% sucrose solution in a ratio of 3:1 often has the same effect as pure 1.8% sucrose solution. It should also be noted that the effect of the hypoosmolar solution used for endothelial cell assessment depends not only on the culture medium applied, but also on the individual cornea. Endothelial cells cannot always be visualized, for example, with hypotonic BSS, but their visualization can then be readily achieved in the same cornea with hypotonic sucrose solution. This phenomenon should be considered in connection with the change of culture medium and the individual cornea. In general the endothelial cells are less clearly recognizable with increased corneal edema, numerous Descemet's membrane folds and strong stromal-epithelial clouding.

We have found that endothelial cells of cooled corneas (e.g. those in short-term culture) could not be visualized well with osmotic stimulation. Prior to light microscopy, corneas should therefore be left at room temperature for a certain period of time.

Time Point of Endothelial Cell Evaluation

Endothelial assessment in organ culture is usually done 3 times during storage of the donor cornea: at the beginning, middle and end of the culture period. Many banks, including ours, restrict microscopy to the beginning and end of the culture period and only perform it in the middle when the initial findings are unclear. Others do the assessment only at the end of the culture period. The most acceptable protocol must be individually determined.

Knowing the condition of the endothelium at the beginning of the culture period helps the examiner to initially assess the quality of a donor cornea and to decide whether culturing is worthwhile. The cornea will not be used for grafting if its initial endothelial cell count is already below the acceptable minimum or if marked endothelial cell necroses are detectable. Moreover, this knowledge will enable an assessment of changes during the culture period. An endothelial cell loss during the culture period is only noted if the endothelial cell density is known at the start.

Endothelial microscopy during culture is best performed halfway through the culture period, e.g. when changing the medium. The condition of the donor cornea after several days of culture is an important point in assessing the probable transplantability. Comparison with the endothelial findings at the start of the culture period enables the detection of changes that occur during its course. For example, marked endothelial cell necroses may indicate bacterial contamination, even if the culture medium does not yet show any changes.

Endothelial assessment at the end of the organ culture determines whether the cornea possesses the quality required for grafting. While an evaluation does not necessarily have to be performed at a different time point like the beginning or middle of organ culture, it is obligatory at the end. For logistic reasons, the final assessment of the corneal endothelium is often done before placing the cornea in dextran-containing deswelling medium. This allows more time for mediating the tissue prior to transplantation. However, we recommend performing the final microscopic assessment only after adequate deswelling. This is the time directly preceding the potential transplantation, and the donor cornea is in the condition in which assessment is most realistic and most reliable. Moreover, since deswelling often induces an endothelial cell loss, previous assessment can yield false high endothelial cell density values. Microscopy of a swollen cornea enables the focusing of only small areas and thus considerably complicates assessment of the endothelial cell layer.

Unlike organ culture, short-term culture (hypothermic storage) is not conducive to regenerative changes due to cold-related cell inhibition. Thus, the condition of the endothelial cell layer will not change during short-term culture. Nevertheless, assessment before and after the culture period should be done here too.

Criteria for Evaluating Endothelium

Three points are important for assessing endothelium: the number, morphology and vitality of the endothelial cells. In the final evaluation of the donor cornea, microscopy should be done in the center, in the 4 paracentral/midperipheral quadrants and in the periphery. After each endothelial evaluation, findings should be documented in detail, preferably together with corresponding endothelial images.

Endothelial Cell Density

The various techniques for determining endothelial cell density are all based on the same principle. The endothelial cells are first microscopically visualized and imaged. Then in a defined area of known size the cells are counted on the image, and the number of endothelial cells per square millimeter are calculated.

Particularly suitable for imaging endothelial cells is a camera coupled to the microscope that captures a live image, e.g. a video or digital camera. The camera image can be displayed on a monitor. It is advisable to use a PC and digitalize the images. The digitalized images can be efficiently stored and processed in different ways, e.g. with special software programs for endothelial cell analysis.

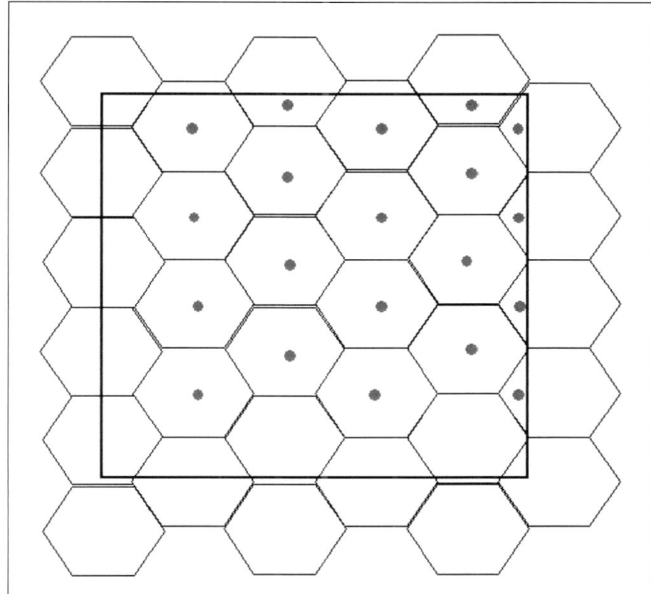

Fig. 2. Schema showing the fixed frame/L method for cell counting; only the cells with the dot are counted for calculating the cell density.

Alternatively, the camera can be coupled directly to a printer for image acquisition. Use of a video recorder to archive findings is also conceivable.

Another way to obtain a microscopic endothelial cell image for counting is to use a still camera. Here an instant camera is preferable to a conventional film camera because of its fast image acquisition. A digital still camera can also be used.

The endothelial cell image is overlaid with a point-counting grid that corresponds to a defined area, taking into account the magnification effects of the lens and camera. For practical purposes, this grid is rectangular with a constant size, and the counting method is thus called the fixed-frame method. The area within the fixed frame is designated as the region of interest (ROI). All cells completely within the grid are counted as well as those touching two adjacent borders. This so-called L method is a simple approach to estimate the number of endothelial cells inside the grid (fig. 2). The cell count thus obtained is then used to calculate the number of endothelial cells per square millimeter of rear corneal surface: cells in the frame (ROI)/frame (ROI) size = cell density/1 mm^2. The cell density is thus obtained by the following formula: [number of cells in the frame (ROI) × 1 mm^2]/frame (ROI) size. This yields, for example, a cell density of 2,000 cells/mm^2 for 100 cells in a frame (ROI) of 0.05 mm^2.

A point-counting grid can easily be created by imaging a Neubauer counting chamber under the same observation conditions used for endothelial cell microscopy. The contours of an area of known size from the microscopic pattern of the counting chamber are transferred to a plastic foil or small glass plate. The grid thus created is then placed on the endothelial cell image, and the cells are counted as described above. It is practical to mark the cells with a pencil to avoid double counting or forgetting any of them. It should be possible to remove these marks from the grid to enable its reuse. This technique of endothelial cell counting is also designated as manual cell counting.

Use of an image analysis system enables computer processing and counting of digitalized endothelial cell images. Special programs are commercially available for use with both a light microscope and a specular microscope (e.g. Navis/Eye Bank by Nidek Technologies, Samba Cornee™ and EAT, Rhine-Tec). Most specular microscopes have integrated software for endothelial cell analysis. Here similar principles are applied for assessing endothelial cells. There are semiautomatic and automatic algorithms. When using a semiautomatic system, the examiner marks endothelial cells with the mouse, and the computer then automatically calculates the endothelial cell density as well as the endothelial cell area and border. Such a widespread method is the so-called center method, where the examiner marks the center of a large number of connected endothelial cells. Calculations are based on the number of points and their distances.

With the automatic programs, the computer independently recognizes single cells and then does calculations based on the number of identified cells and their areas. Automatic single-cell detection is strongly dependent on the quality of endothelial cell visualization and is thus highly susceptible to errors. Automatic cell recognition usually requires manual processing to obtain correct results.

Only one system, the Navis/Eye Bank software (Nidek Technologies), currently enables fully automatic estimation of endothelial cell density without single-cell recognition. An endothelial cell image magnified 100-fold is submitted to frequency analysis, and thus endothelial cell density is determined in about 1 s. This technique was found to show high conformity with manual determination of endothelial cell density by the fixed-frame method [7].

Apart from providing easy, inexpensive and efficient image acquisition and archiving, the use of software for endothelial cell analysis offers the advantage of an endothelial cell assessment superior to that achieved by purely manual cell counting. Thus, the computer-based fixed-frame/L method, for example, already has the advantage of enabling the analysis of very large areas.

Irrespective of the counting method, the correct size of the counting grid is essential for reliable endothelial cell counting. Thus, it is imperative to check and possibly adjust this if there are changes in the microscope or the attached camera. In addition, calibration of the counting grid should be routinely checked from time to time. Faulty calibration of the counting grid has proved to be the most frequent cause of false endothelial cell counts [8].

A simple method for estimating the cell count during light microscopy is to use an eyepiece with a counting grid. When used by examiners with adequate experience, it is easy to perform and quickly yields relatively precise estimations of the endothelial cell count. Thus, it is well suited for endothelial assessment before and during the culture period. We feel it is too imprecise for the final endothelial evaluation at the end of culture because of the very small counted area of about 0.01 mm^2 and the lack of endothelial cell images.

To estimate the endothelial cell count in donor eyes prior to preparation, a non-contact specular microscope (e.g. Noncon Robo Specular Microscope SP 6000, Konan Medical Inc.; Endothel Kamera SP-3000, Topcon) can be used as in the patient examination. The intact donor eyeball is held in front of the camera with one hand under sterile conditions, and the apparatus is operated with the other hand.

In general, we recommend a minimum cell count of 100/frame (ROI) for calculating the cell density. The higher the number of counted cells, the more precise the calculated cell density. Because of physiological variation, it is useful to determine the cell density in different central corneal areas and to calculate an average value. The more irregular the cell pattern (e.g. high polymegathism), the higher the cell count should be in order to avoid overestimating the cell density.

Good cell visibility/image quality is necessary for reliable cell counting. Frequently only a small endothelial area is visible when corneas are examined in a swollen condition, and that area is diagonal to the observation axis. These factors easily lead to a false high endothelial cell density in swollen corneas.

An adequately high endothelial cell density after the culture period is a decisive criterion that must be met before releasing a donor cornea for grafting. An endothelial cell density of 2,000–2,200 cells/mm^2 is generally recognized as the lower limit for the longest possible graft survival [9]. Clear graft survival in the recipient is highly dependent on the endothelial cell density. Irreversible graft clouding often occurs if the density is below the critical limit of about 400 cells/mm^2. Corneal grafting may be assumed to entail an endothelial cell loss of about 10% due to mechanical forces. In the posttransplantation period, the endothelial cell loss is markedly accelerated (about 7- to 15-fold) compared to that associated with natural corneal aging [10]. Viewed statistically, at least 1 endothelial cell/mm^2 is lost each day. Thus, a correctly determined and adequately high endothelial cell density is extremely important for the graft recipient.

Endothelial Cell Vitality

The endothelial cell density decreases by about 10% during the culture period [11]. Manipulation during removal and preparation is probably a major cause. An endothelial cell loss is surely also caused by nutrient deficiency or unphysiological conditions of the culture medium. In addition, an important role is played by changes in corneal metabolism related to the duration of culture. During organ culture, necrotic cells detach from the cell layer and assume a spherical shape. These dead cells are then recognizable over the endothelial cell layer even without osmotic stimulation.

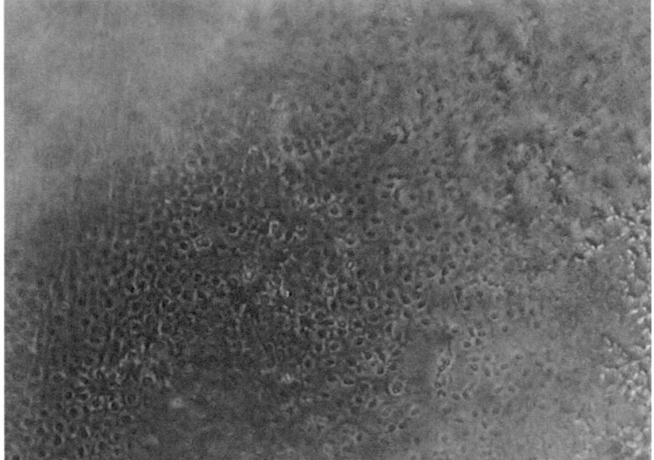

Fig. 3. Detached and necrotic endothelial cells, on the right side some vital endothelial cells which respond to the osmotic stimulation. Hypotonic BSS, inverse microscope with phase contrast technique. Magnification ×200.

Light microscopy of a cornea in culture medium thus enables simple estimation of the degree of endothelial cell necroses. The necrotic endothelial cells may be disseminated over the entire endothelial surface area or coherently affect larger areas. Such marked necroses are microscopically visualized as a confluently detached cell sheet (fig. 3). While the gaps caused by single cell necroses are closed by vital adjacent endothelial cells, Descemet's membrane is denuded by extensive necroses. Single necroses often occur more frequently near Descemet's folds induced by corneal swelling in culture medium or mechanical forces.

Recognition of devitalized cells is facilitated by vital staining, which is the technique of staining living cells without causing dye-induced structural changes or damage. Trypan blue has long been used effectively for this purpose and leads to intensive blue staining of the nuclei of membrane-damaged cells and denuded Descemet's membrane. Vital cells with an intact cell membrane remain unstained [12] (fig. 4). Trypan blue staining is very easy to perform. The donor cornea is removed from the culture medium, rinsed with BSS to remove remaining medium and placed endothelium side up on a sterile surface (e.g. BD Falcon cell culture dish 35 × 10 mm). One to two drops of sterile isotonic trypan blue solution are put on the endothelial side. After about 45 s, the cornea is grasped with sterile forceps at the scleral rim; the staining solution is then shaken off, and the cornea is rinsed with BSS to remove the remaining trypan blue. Larger areas of connected endothelial cell necroses and denuded Descemet's membrane would then show strong blue staining and would already be clearly visible to the naked eye. Slight staining of the scleral rim is usually unavoidable but harmless. After trypan blue staining, single cell necroses have blue-stained nuclei and are thus easily recognized by light microscopy.

The advantage of trypan blue staining is the simplicity and reliability with which devitalized endothelial cells can be visualized. It may be helpful in cases where corneal

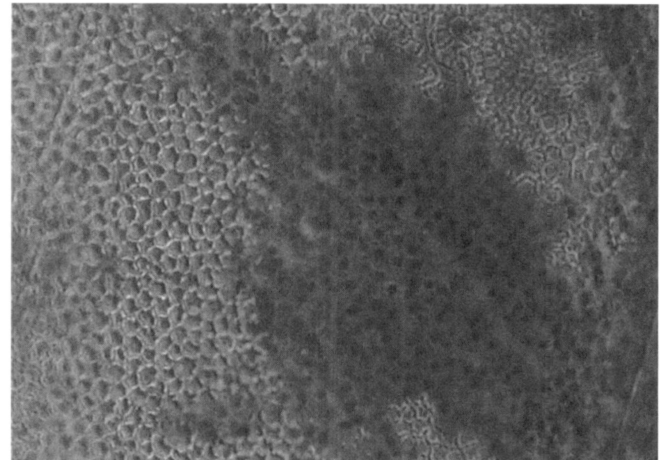

Fig. 4. Endothelium of a human donor cornea before organ culture with a large area of necrotic cells with blue nuclei after trypan blue staining. Hypotonic BSS, inverse microscope with phase contrast technique. Magnification ×200.

edema prevents fast microscopic examination of the entire endothelial cell layer. If the entire layer can be microscopically visualized and morphologically assessed, trypan blue staining will not yield additional information.

Trypan blue is commercially available as a sterile isotonic solution, also in premixed preparations for use in the eye during surgical interventions (Vision Blue™, Dorc; TB-S, Alchimia Srl). The dye is also available as a dry substance, and sterile preparations can be self-mixed and bottled, but attention must be paid to the osmolarity and pH value of the finished solution. Data from various cornea banks disclose an applied concentration of 0.2–0.5% and an exposure time of 30–90 s (European Eye Bank Association Directory). Trypan blue has a concentration- and time-dependent toxic effect in the range of a solution exceeding 1% and an exposure time of several minutes. No noxious influence is to be expected with the protocol described above.

Vital staining of the corneal endothelium with fluorescein diacetate (FDA) is another technique for vitality analysis [13]. In contrast to trypan blue, which selectively stains damaged cells, FDA can visualize actively metabolizing vital cells. FDA solution (1 mg/ml), which is not toxic to the endothelium, is dripped onto the endothelial side and removed by rinsing with an isotonic buffer solution (e.g. BSS) after 5–10 s. However, the staining results can only be seen under a fluorescence microscope (stimulation at a wavelength of 430 nm). The yellowish green fluorescent endothelial cells can be clearly distinguished from dark areas in the cell layer corresponding to devitalized or damaged cells. Metabolic degradation of the dye leads to decreasing fluorescence intensity, and thus analysis is only possible for about 30 min. However, FDA staining has not yet become generally accepted in the clinical routine.

A simple and reliable test for the biological quality and health of endothelial cells is not yet available for cultured corneas. Good visualization of endothelial cells and their susceptibility to the influence of osmotically active substances are still the best signs of vitality. The failure to visualize endothelial cell borders by hypoosmolar substances and an accelerated cell loss during organ culture indicate poor quality of the cornea.

Endothelial cell necroses influence the donor cornea quality in proportion to the extent and localization of the defect as well as the vital endothelial cell density. A rule of thumb here is: the more peripheral and smaller the necrosis and the higher the endothelial cell density, the more insignificant the necrotic area. Central multicell or group necroses often lead to the loss of a donor cornea.

Endothelial Cell Morphology

Endothelial cells often show deviations from their typical hexagonality. Morphology assessment should routinely involve estimating the pleomorphism (deviation from hexagonality), polymegathism (variation in cell area) and granulation/vacuolization of the endothelial cells.

Apart from cell density, regularity of the endothelium is an important point in evaluating the suitability of donor corneas for grafting. A high degree of polymegathism and pleomorphism is regarded a negative sign, though little is known about the influence of these changes on endothelial cell function or corneal graft survival. High polymegathism and pleomorphism and low cell density are associated with low functional quality of the corneal endothelium.

Since the human corneal endothelial cell layer is a postmitotic tissue, cell loss leads to enlargement and migration of the remaining cells and thus to increased polymegathism and pleomorphism. Hence all factors causing cell loss (e.g. aging, hypoxia, mechanical stress to the cornea, Descemet's membrane folds and endothelial wounding) also cause an increase in polymegathism and pleomorphism. This is a typical phenomenon in organ-cultured corneas, where significant cell loss, especially in areas of Descemet's membrane folds, causes obvious morphological changes in the endothelial cell layer (fig. 5). High polymegathism and pleomorphism are more frequent in corneas with low endothelial cell densities. In short-term culture (hypothermic storage), no change of endothelial cell morphology is to be expected during the culture period due to the lack of regenerative processes.

Several indices have been reported for the description of polymegathism and pleomorphism. The one most frequently used for polymegathism is the coefficient of variation. Here the calculated standard deviation of an endothelial cell sample is related to the calculated average cell area (standard deviation/mean cell area). The coefficient of variation can also be expressed as a percentage: (standard deviation/mean cell area) × 100.

Pleomorphism can be expressed in terms of polygonality (number of neighboring cells) and hexagonality (percentage of hexagonal cells).

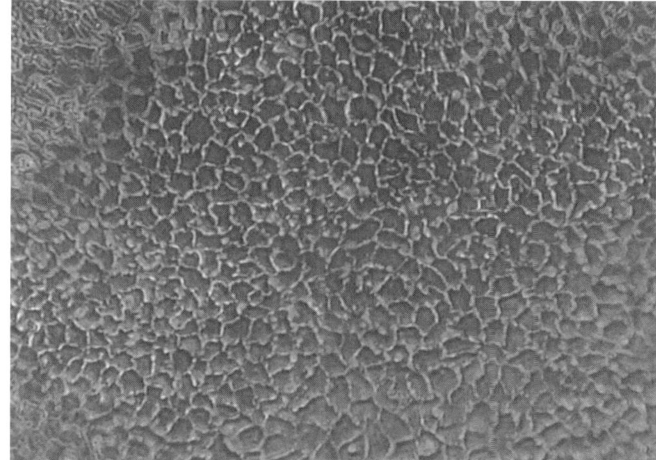

Fig. 5. Endothelium with significant polymegathism and pleomorphism of a human donor cornea after organ culture. Hypotonic BSS, inverse microscope with phase contrast technique. Magnification ×200.

Precise determination of the polymegathism and pleomorphism of endothelial cells is difficult and can only be done with the aid of special computer programs. The exact size measurement and cell side detection of many single cells are necessary for a precise estimation of the polymegathism and pleomorphism. The center method is a simpler approach for determining these parameters. After manual labeling of cell centers, the computer program calculates polymegathism from the varying distances of cell centers and pleomorphism from the number of neighboring cells. It is much easier to grade the regularity of endothelial cells by having an experienced investigator examine the image. So far this is the most common method for assessing polymegathism and pleomorphism of the endothelium in eye banking.

It should be kept in mind that the osmotic stimulation needed for light microscopy but not for specular microscopy artificially changes the cell image. Thus, changes caused by osmotic stimulation (e.g. vacuolization induced by 1.8% sucrose solution) must be distinguished from true morphological changes.

Apart from morphological changes in the endothelial cells themselves, there are other pathological or degenerative changes in the endothelial cell layer that have to be considered in microscopy or slitlamp biomicroscopy. Protein deposits, inflammatory cells and pigment are often seen as the result of intraocular inflammation or pigment dispersion. Corneal endothelial cells can phagocytize pigment; for example, iris pigment may thus be deposited in these cells. Defects in Descemet's membrane caused for example by cataract surgery can be easily recognized and stained with trypan blue.

Particular attention should be given to the presence of guttae, i.e. wart-like excrescences on Descemet's membrane. Guttae are visualized by light microscopy as round structures about the same size as endothelial cells (fig. 6). They resemble

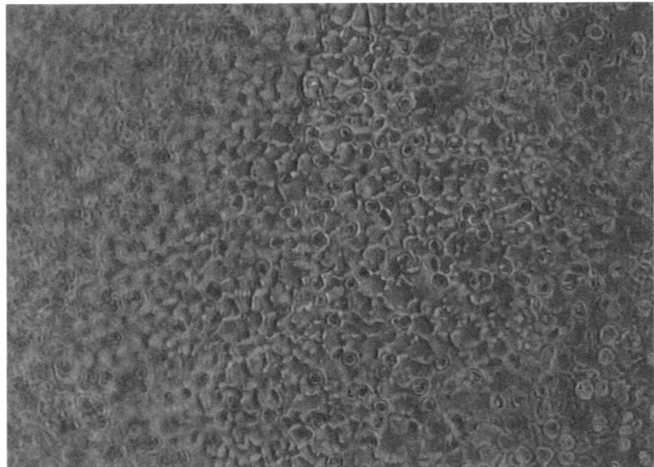

Fig. 6. Human cornea endothelium with a high number of guttae. Hypotonic BSS, inverse microscope with phase contrast technique. Magnification ×200.

single cell necroses but can be distinguished from them by their localization on the endothelial cell surface and not above it. In specular microscopy, guttae appear as round black spots in the endothelial cell layer. When examined by splitlamp biomicroscopy, guttae make the endothelial cell layer look like hammered metal with tiny round gaps between the endothelial cells and are thus relatively easy to recognize at higher magnification (e.g. 32-fold). Guttae are accompanied by a loss of endothelial cells, and an increased postoperative endothelial cell loss has been demonstrated for corneal grafts with these changes [14]. The described pathological changes, particularly the presence of guttae, render a donor cornea unsuitable for grafting.

Hassall-Henle warts or bodies are regarded as harmless changes related to physiological aging of the endothelial cell layer. These round wart-like elevations on the posterior surface of Descemet's membrane are found at the periphery of the cornea, whereas guttae develop at the center.

Experimental Endothelial Staining

Trypan Blue and Alizarin Red S Sequential Staining

Because of its simplicity, this combination stain has long been used for clinicopathological and experimental examinations of corneas. While trypan blue stains the nuclei of devitalized cells, alizarin red intensively marks the cell membrane. The endothelial cell borders are thus clearly visible (fig. 7). Alizarin red S is cytotoxic and causes irreversible endothelial cell damage. This renders the stain unsuitable for donor corneas destined to be grafted [15, 16].

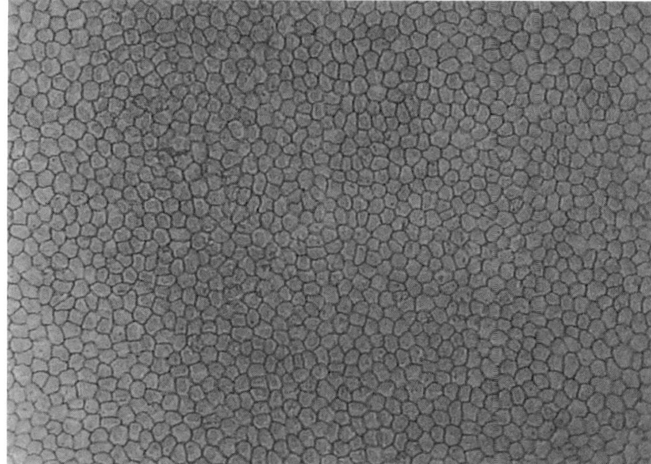

Fig. 7. Porcine endothelium after alizarin red S stain. Inverse microscope. Magnification ×200.

Staining Procedure

Trypan blue is used as a preparation of a 0.25% solution in physiological sodium chloride.

Alizarin red S (alizarin sulfonic acid sodium) is prepared as a 0.2% solution in physiological sodium chloride solution. Alizarin red is not freely soluble in water and must be dissolved for several hours with the magnetic stirrer and filtrated before use. The pH value of the solution thus prepared is adjusted to 4.2 using 0.1% sodium chloride solution (approx. 250 ml/10 ml of solution) [17].

First the cornea is stained with trypan blue as described above. After rinsing to remove the dye, alizarin red S solution is applied to the endothelial side and poured off after about 90 s and thoroughly rinsed with isotonic electrolyte solution. Since staining results vary after alizarin red S, shorter or longer exposure times may be needed. All cell nuclei are visualized when trypan blue staining is repeated after applying 99% ethanol.

Alizarin red S staining can also be performed independently of trypan blue staining and visualizes the cell borders without osmotic changes. It is thus well suited for learning and perfecting endothelial assessment. It is easy to perform alizarin red S staining after vital microscopy with osmotic stimulation and to thus get a feeling for the different visualizations of endothelial cells.

Janus Green Photometry Technique

The Janus green photometry technique is based on rapid and complete extraction of the basic vital dye Janus green from the stained cornea. The amount of dye extracted corresponds to the degree of endothelial damage. The endothelial alteration can be directly determined by photometric measurement of the elution solution and transfer of the extinction value to a standard curve. The extracted dye solution can be stored for weeks until measurement. This technique offers an in vitro alternative to the usual time-consuming procedure of counting stained cells. It is well suited for experimental analysis of endothelial damage, caused for example by intraocular rinsing solutions, surgical techniques and corneal culture media. A detailed description of the Janus green photometry technique can be found in the literature cited [18].

References

1 Waring GO, Bourne WM, Edelhauser HF, Kenyon KR: The corneal endothelium: normal and pathologic structure and function. Ophthalmology 1982; 89:531–590.

2 Shamsuddin AK, Nirankari VS, Purnell DM, Chang SH: Is the corneal posterior cell layer truly endothelial? Ophthalmology 1986;93:1298–1303.

3 Schimmelpfennig BH: Direct and indirect determination of nonuniform cell density distribution in human corneal endothelium. Invest Ophthalmol Vis Sci 1984;25:223–229.

4 Leber T: Studien über den Flüssigkeitswechsel im Auge. Albrecht von Graefe's Arch Ophthalmol 1883; 19:7–181.

5 Fischberg J, Hernandez J, Liebovitch LS, Koniarek JP: The mechanism of fluid and electrolyte transport across corneal endothelium: critical revision and update of a model. Curr Eye Res 1985;4:351–360.

6 Meltendorf C, Ohrloff C, Rieck P, Schroeter J: Endothelial cell density in porcine corneas after exposure to hypotonic solutions. Graefes Arch Clin Exp Ophthalmol 2007;245:143–147.

7 Ruggeri A, Grisan E, Jaroszewski J: A new system for the automatic estimation of endothelial cell density in donor corneas. Br J Ophthalmol 2005;89:306–311.

8 Thuret G, Manissolle C, Acquart S, Le Petit JC, Maugery J, Campos-Guyotat L, Doughty MJ, Gain P: Is manual counting of corneal endothelial cell density in eye banks still acceptable? The French experience. Br J Ophthalmol 2003;12:1481–1486.

9 Armitage WJ, Dick AD, Bourne WM: Predicting endothelial cell loss and long-term corneal graft survival. Invest Ophthalmol Vis Sci 2003;44:3326–3331.

10 Bourne WM, Hodge DO, Nelson LR: Corneal endothelium five years after transplantation. Am J Ophthalmol 1994;118:185–196.

11 Pels, E, Schuchard Y: Organ-culture preservation of human corneas. Doc Ophthalmol 1983;56:147–153.

12 Sperling S: Evaluation of the endothelium of human donor corneas by induced dilation of intercellular spaces and trypan blue. Graefes Arch Clin Exp Ophthalmol 1986;224:428–434.

13 Wilhelm, F, Melzig M, Franke G: Vital staining by fluorescein diacetate (FDA) – a method for estimation of corneal endothelium. Acta Ophthalmol 1990;68:94–96.

14 Borderie VM, Sabolic V, Touzeau O, Scheer S, Carvajal-Gonzalez S, Laroche L: Screening human donor corneas during organ culture for the presence of guttae. Br J Ophthalmol 2003;87:515–516.

15 Sperling S: Combined staining of corneal endothelium by alizarin red and trypan blue. Acta Ophthalmol 1977;55:573–580.

16 Spence DJ, Peyman GA: A new technique for the vital staining of corneal endothelium. Invest Ophthalmol Vis Sci 1976;15:1000–1002.

17 Taylor MJ, Hunt CJ: Dual staining of corneal endothelium with trypan blue and alizarin red S: importance of pH for the dye-lake reaction. Br J Ophthalmol 1981;65:815–819.

18 Hartmann C, Rieck P: A new test for endothelial viability: the Janus green photometry technique. Arch Ophthalmol 1989;107:1511–1515.

Jan Schroeter
Cornea Bank Berlin, Department of Ophthalmology, Charité – Universitätsmedizin Berlin, Campus-Virchow-Klinikum
Augustenburger Platz 1
DE–13353 Berlin (Germany)
Tel. +49 0 30 450 554 099, Fax +49 0 30 450 554 989, E-Mail jan.schroeter@charite.de

Bredehorn-Mayr T, Duncker GIW, Armitage WJ (eds): Eye Banking.
Dev Ophthalmol. Basel, Karger, 2009, vol 43, pp 63–69

Cryopreservation for Corneal Storage

W. John Armitage

Department of Clinical Science, University of Bristol, Bristol, UK

Abstract

Currently, cryopreservation is the only method that offers the prospect of truly long-term storage of living cells and tissues. Despite some successful cryopreserved corneal grafts, freezing has been shown to damage the endothelium. When isolated cells are frozen, there are two principal mechanisms of damage: intracellular freezing, which occurs at high cooling rates, and solution effect injury at low cooling rates. When tissues are frozen, there are additional factors that appear to render cells more susceptible to intracellular freezing. Lower cooling rates appear to overcome this when freezing cornea. Vitrification is a way of achieving ice-free cryopreservation, but it also poses considerable challenges owing to the very high solute concentrations required to achieve vitrification at practicable cooling rates. Encouraging results have also been reported for cornea frozen using non-permeating cryoprotectants, which could lead to simpler methods of corneal cryopreservation.

Cryopreservation offers the prospect of truly long-term storage of living cells and tissues. A number of successful full-thickness grafts were carried out with cryopreserved corneas in the 1960s and 1970s using the methods developed independently by O'Neill et al. [1] in the UK and Capella et al. [2] in the USA. The initial graft survival was somewhat lower than would be expected today, and the corneas took rather longer to clear. It was therefore suggested that the usefulness of these methods was limited to corneas from young donors (presumably with high endothelial cell densities) cryopreserved within just a few hours of death, although this was later disputed [3]. The methods were shown to cause damage, especially to the endothelium [4, 5], yet some cryopreserved grafts did achieve long-term survival [6]. Despite the universal application of hypothermia and organ culture for storing corneas and the view that cryopreservation was overly complex for routine application in eye banks, there are a few eye banks that still use cryopreservation to store tissue for emergency grafts [7] or for storing non-viable tissue for anterior lamellar or tectonic grafts [8]. Research continues into the mechanisms of corneal cryo-injury, especially to the endothelium, not only to develop improved methods of corneal cryopreservation, but also because the cornea provides a valuable model system for other organized tissues and tissue-engineered constructs.

Freezing Injury

When a suspension of cells is cooled, ice initially forms outside the cells in the surrounding medium. The crystallization of ice effectively removes pure water from the suspending medium, causing a rise in solute concentration. As more ice forms with falling temperature, there is a corresponding and substantial concentration of solutes. The fate of cells exposed to these conditions depends largely on the rate of cooling [9, 10]. Owing to the semipermeable properties of the plasma membrane, a rise in external solute concentration causes a passive efflux of water from cells, thereby maintaining osmotic equilibrium. When the cooling rate is low, the cell loses water in response to the rise in external solute concentration resulting in extremely shrunken cells surrounded by extracellular ice. At higher cooling rates, however, the cells cannot lose water rapidly enough to maintain osmotic equilibrium, the cytoplasm supercools below its freezing point until thermodynamic equilibrium is eventually restored by intracellular freezing [11]. The cells are consequently much less shrunken compared with slowly cooled cells but they contain ice, which is usually lethal [12].

When cell survival is plotted as a function of cooling rate, a maximum is typically observed at an optimum cooling rate with survival falling at higher or lower cooling rates, which suggests that there are two mechanisms of freezing injury [10]. This is illustrated in figure 1 where the cells frozen in suspension show an optimum cooling rate of 1°C/min. At rates higher than the optimum, the cells are damaged as a consequence of intracellular freezing, but at lower rates, the mechanism of damage is related to prolonged exposure to the very high electrolyte concentrations (i.e. solution effects or slow cooling injury) [14]. The rate of warming can also have a marked influence on cell survival [15].

Cryoprotectants

Most cells do not survive freezing and thawing unless a cryoprotectant is used. A wide range of compounds have cryoprotective properties, but glycerol [16] and dimethyl sulphoxide [17], which both permeate cells, are among the most efficient and widely used cryoprotectants. Cryoprotectants are effective against slow cooling injury but do not protect cells against damage from intracellular ice. Consequently, with increasing initial concentration of cryoprotectant, survival increases and the optimum cooling rate shifts to lower values [18].

However, cryoprotectants can themselves be harmful to cells due to chemical toxicity and osmotic stress during their addition to and removal from cells. Since plasma

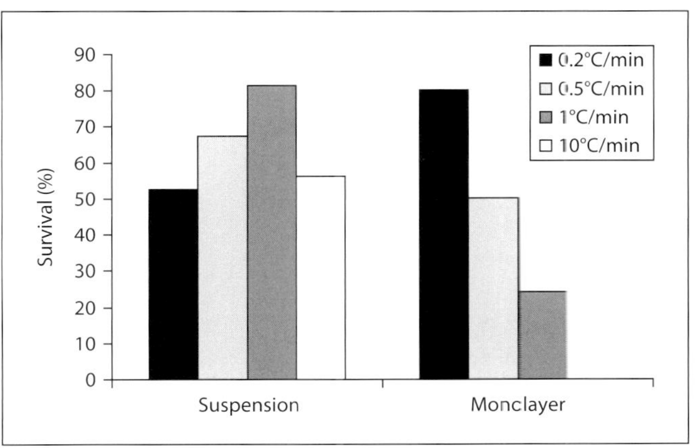

Fig. 1. Effect of cooling rate on survival of keratocytes after freezing and thawing either in suspension or as monolayers. Cells were cooled at 0.2, 0.5, 1 or 10°C/min in 10% (v/v) propane-1,2-diol. Note lower optimum cooling rate in monolayers and marked fall in survival with increasing cooling rate. Redrawn from Armitage and Juss [13] with publisher's permission.

membranes are more permeable to water than to cryoprotectants, abrupt changes in external concentration of such a permeating solute causes transient changes in cell volume as water moves rapidly across the membrane to restore osmotic equilibrium followed by a slower return to normal cell volume as the solute permeates down its concentration gradient [19, 20]. During addition of cryoprotectant, cells initially shrink before returning to normal volume, but an abrupt reduction in external cryoprotectant concentration during its removal by dilution can cause substantial cell swelling. Most cells tolerate shrinkage better than swelling, although some are also damaged by relatively small amounts of shrinkage [21, 22]. When cells swell, damage occurs even before the lytic volume is reached, leaving cells with an apparently intact plasma membrane yet functionally damaged. This is one of the reasons why membrane integrity assays of cell survival need to be interpreted with caution. Swelling can be limited by diluting the cryoprotectant in steps or by adding a non-permeating solute to act as an osmotic buffer [23]. For cells that are sensitive to shrinkage, the cryoprotectant may also need to be added in steps. Corneal endothelium appears to be relatively tolerant of osmotic stress [24].

Some non-permeating sugars, proteins and polymers also have cryoprotective properties, but they tend to be less effective than permeating cryoprotectants. They do, however, have the advantage of avoiding the osmotic stress associated with the use of permeating cryoprotectants, and compounds such as dextran have been investigated for corneal cryopreservation with encouraging results [25, 26].

Freezing Injury in Tissues

Unlike a suspension of cells, tissues tend to have a fixed geometry and mass, which limits the range of cooling and warming rates that can be applied. In this respect, the size and shape of the cornea are not such a barrier as when freezing larger tissues and organs.

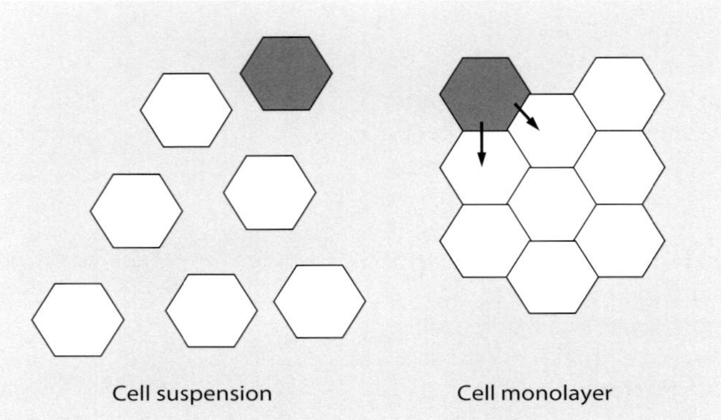

Fig. 2. Consequences of intracellular freezing (dark cells) in isolated cell suspension or in cell monolayers where there is potential for the spread of ice between neighbouring cells.

Tissues contain a range of cells, each with its own optimum cooling rate; but this factor becomes less important at higher cryoprotectant concentrations. On the other hand, other factors such as high density of cells and the presence of cell junctions may render cells in organized structures more susceptible to freezing injury than isolated cells [27]. Figure 1 compares the cooling rate dependence of survival of corneal keratocytes when frozen in 10% (v/v) propane-1,2-diol as isolated cells in suspension or as monolayers [13]. Isolated cells achieved 80% survival at an optimum cooling rate of 1°C/min. At the same cooling rate, only 25% of cells in monolayers survived. Reducing the cooling rate to just 0.2°C/min increased survival in the monolayers to 80% but reduced survival of isolated cells to 50%. The steep decrease in survival in the monolayers with increasing cooling rate indicated a greater susceptibility to intracellular freezing, perhaps by the spread of intracellular ice through gap junctions to neighbouring cells [28, 29]. On the other hand, if a single cell in a dispersed suspension freezes, it is an isolated event that has no impact on other cells (fig. 2). The data in figure 1 also suggest that cells in monolayers are more tolerant of slow cooling injury than isolated cells.

The corneal cryopreservation methods developed in the 1960s used cooling rates between 1 and 5°C/min. These rates, at least for the rabbit cornea, cause severe damage to the endothelium, suggesting that human and dog corneas are more tolerant of freezing. Since corneal endothelial cells are interconnected by gap junctions, the potential exists for the spread of intracellular ice between cells. Reducing the cooling rate of rabbit corneas to 0.2°C/min has been shown to improve endothelial structural and functional survival, which supports this concept [30].

Vitrification

To avoid the mechanisms of freezing injury, ice-free cryopreservation by vitrification has been explored for a range of cells and tissues, including cornea [31,

32]. Freezing and vitrification both describe the solidification of liquids brought about by cooling, but the mechanisms are entirely different [33]. When a solution freezes, water undergoes a phase transition from liquid to crystalline solid (ice), causing a substantial rise in solute concentration. During vitrification, crystallization is suppressed by an extreme elevation in viscosity of the solution. The solution takes on the physical properties of a solid at the glass transition temperature when the viscosity reaches approximately 10^{14} Pa•s, yet the molecules remain randomly arranged as in a liquid. As there is no crystallization of ice, there is no phase separation of water and solute and therefore no rise in solute concentration during cooling.

To achieve this amorphous state requires extremely high cooling rates, far higher than could be achieved for cornea. Fortunately, the addition of solutes such as cryoprotectants raises the viscosity of the solution, increases glass transition temperature and lowers the critical cooling rate needed to vitrify. However, the cryoprotectant concentrations required are 5- to 10-fold higher than would be required in their conventional role as protectors against freezing injury, and this is a significant barrier to this approach to cryopreservation.

Vitrification solutions often consist of complex mixtures of cryoprotectants and other solutes in order to try to minimize the toxicity of individual components. Embryos and vascular tissue have been vitrified using such solutions [34, 35], but this approach has not thus far been successful for cornea [36]. However, functional survival of endothelium has been reported after vitrification of rabbit corneas at –110°C in a solution containing 6.8 mol/l propane-1,2-diol, which has efficient glass-forming properties [37]. This is a higher concentration than is needed to vitrify but was necessary to avoid devitrification, which is the crystallization of ice during warming [33]. This method is currently too complex and time consuming for routine eye banking taking 90 and 60 min, respectively, to add and remove the vitrification solution, but the results at least support the feasibility of vitrifying corneas.

Cryopreservation – The Future

In summary, attempts to cryopreserve corneas for penetrating keratoplasty have met with varying degrees of success. Despite some successful grafts in patients in the 1960s and 1970s, cryopreservation was shown to inflict significant endothelial damage, although this did not preclude the long-term survival of some cryopreserved grafts. Cryopreservation has since continued to be investigated, bringing a better understanding of the mechanisms of endothelial injury and the development of new methodologies such as vitrification and freezing with non-permeating cryoprotectants. If a reliable, simplified method can be achieved, cryopreservation may yet find wider application in eye banking.

References

1 O'Neill P, Mueller FO, Trevor-Roper PD: On the preservation of corneae at –196°C for full-thickness homografts in man and dog. Br J Ophthalmoly 1967;51:13–30.
2 Capella JA, Kaufman HE, Robbins JE: Preservation of viable corneal tissue. Cryobiology 1965;2:116–121.
3 Ehlers N, Sperling S, Olsen T: Post-operative thickness and endothelial cells density in cultivated cryopreserved human corneal grafts. Acta Ophthalmol 1982;60:935–944.
4 Van Horn DL, Hanna C, Schultz RO: Corneal cryopreservation. II. Ultrastructural and viability changes. Arch Ophthalmol 1970;84:655–667.
5 Van Horn DL, Schultz RO: Endothelial survival in cryopreserved human corneas: a scanning electron microscope study. Invest Ophthalmol Vis Sci 1974; 13:7–16.
6 Schultz RO, Matsuda M, Yee RW, Glasser DB, Sabin SM, Edelhauser HF: Long-term survival of cryopreserved corneal endothelium. Ophthalmology 1985; 92:1663–1667.
7 Brunette I, Le François M, Tremblay MC, Guertin MC: Corneal transplant tolerance of cryopreservation. Cornea 2001;20:590–596.
8 Yao Y-F, Zhang Y-M, Zhou P, Zhang B, Qiu W-Y, Tseng SCG: Therapeutic penetrating keratoplasty in severe fungal keratitis using cryopreserved corneas. Cornea 2003;87:543–547.
9 Mazur P: Freezing of living cells: mechanisms and implications. Am J Physiol 1984;247:C125–C142.
10 Mazur P: Cryobiology: the freezing of biological systems. Science 1970;168:939–949.
11 Mazur P: Kinetics of water loss from cells at subzero temperatures and the likelihood of intracellular freezing. J Gen Physiol 1963;47:347–369.
12 Mazur P: The role of intracellular freezing in the death of cells cooled at supraoptimal rates. Cryobiology 1977;14:251–272.
13 Armitage WJ, Juss BK: The influence of cooling rate on survival of frozen cells differs in monolayers and in suspensions. Cryoletters 1996;17:213–218.
14 Lovelock JE: The haemolysis of human red bloodcells by freezing and thawing. Biochim Biophys Acta 1953;10:414–426.
15 Miller RH, Mazur P: Survival of frozen-thawed human red cells as a function of cooling and warming velocities. Cryobiology 1976;13:404–414.
16 Polge C, Smith AU, Parkes AS: Revival of spermatozoa after vitrification and dehydration at low temperatures. Nature 1949;164:666.
17 Lovelock JE, Bishop MWH: Prevention of freezing damage to living cells by dimethyl sulphoxide. Nature 1959;183:1394–1395.
18 Leibo SP, Farrant J, Mazur P, Hanna MG Jr, Smith LH: Effects of freezing on marrow stem cell suspensions: interactions of cooling and warming rates in the presence of PVP, sucrose, or glycerol. Cryobiology 1970;6:315–332.
19 House CR: Water Transport in Cells and Tissues. London, Arnold, 1974.
20 Kleinhans FW: Membrane permeability modeling: Kedem-Katchalsky vs a two-parameter formalism. Cryobiology 1998;37:271–289.
21 Armitage WJ, Mazur P: Osmotic tolerance of human granulocytes. Am J Physiol 1984;247:C373–C381.
22 Armitage WJ, Parmar N, Hunt CJ: The effects of osmotic stress on human platelets. J Cell Physiol 1985;123:241–248.
23 Armitage WJ: Osmotic stress as a factor in the detrimental effect of glycerol on human platelets. Cryobiology 1986;23:116–125.
24 Armitage WJ, Moss SJ, Easty DL: Effects of osmotic stress on rabbit corneal endothelium. Cryobiology 1988;25:425–439.
25 Halberstadt M, Athmann S, Hagenah M: Corneal cryopreservation with dextran. Cryobiology 2001; 43:71–80.
26 Halberstadt M, Bohnke M, Athmann S, Hagenah M: Cryopreservation of human donor corneas with dextran. Invest Ophthalmol Vis Sci 2003;44:5110–5115.
27 Taylor MJ, Pegg DE: The effect of ice formation on the function of smooth muscle tissue stored at –21 or –60°C. Cryobiology 1983;20:36–40.
28 Berger WK, Uhrik B: Freeze-induced shrinkage of individual cells and cell-to-cell propagation of intracellular ice in cell chains from salivary glands. Experientia 1996;52:843–850.
29 Acker JP, Elliott JA, McGann LE: Intercellular ice propagation: experimental evidence for ice growth through membrane pores. Biophys J 2001;81:1389–1397.
30 Routledge C, Armitage WJ: Cryopreservation of cornea: a low cooling rate improves functional survival of endothelium after freezing and thawing. Cryobiology 2003;46:277–283.
31 Fahy GM, MacFarlane DR, Angell CA, Meryman HT: Vitrification as an approach to cryopreservation. Cryobiology 1984;21:407–426.
32 Armitage WJ, Rich SJ: Vitrification of organized tissues. Cryobiology 1990;27:483–491.
33 MacFarlane DR: Physical aspects of vitrification in aqueous solutions. Cryobiology 1987;24:181–195.
34 Rall WF, Fahy GM: Ice-free cryopreservation of mouse embryos at –196°C by vitrification. Nature 1985;313:573–575.

35 Song YC, Khirabadi BS, Lightfoot F, Brockbank KG, Taylor MJ: Vitreous cryopreservation maintains the function of vascular grafts. Nat Biotechnol 2000;18:296–299.

36 Bourne WM, Nelson LR: Human corneal studies with a vitrification solution containing dimethyl sulfoxide, formamide, and 1,2-propanediol. Cryobiology 1994;31:522–530.

37 Armitage WJ, Hall SC, Routledge C: Recovery of endothelial function after vitrification of cornea at –110°C. Invest Ophthalmol Vis Sci 2002;43:2160–2164.

Prof. W.J. Armitage
University of Bristol, Bristol Eye Hospital
Lower Maudlin Street
Bristol BS1 2LX (UK)
Tel. +44 0 117 928 4585, Fax +44 0 117 904 6624, E-Mail w.j.armitage@bristol.ac.uk

Bredehorn-Mayr T, Duncker GIW, Armitage WJ (eds): Eye Banking.
Dev Ophthalmol. Basel, Karger, 2009, vol 43, pp 70–86

Quality Management in European Eye Banks

Mauro Toniolo · Davide Camposampiero · Carlo Griffoni · Gary L.A. Jones

Fondazione Banca degli Occhi del Veneto, Venice, Italy

Abstract

Background: The European Directive on setting standards of quality and safety for human tissues and cells obliges tissue establishments to implement a quality management system (QMS), based on the principles of good practice, in order to assure a high level of protection with regard to the health of recipients of human tissues. **Methods:** A systematic approach to quality management should be used and sustained. Although a number of quality systems can be employed, a recommended reference model is the ISO 9001:2000 standard which is particularly relevant to eye banking as it can be implemented to cover the entire donation-transplantation process to ensure that the tissues distributed, and services offered, by eye banks show uniform safety and quality. **Results:** The adoption and correct management of a QMS is essential to maximise the benefits and minimise the risks for all those involved in the process. The performance and results of this system must be monitored and measured by appropriate parameters/indicators (positive and negative) which pertain to the structure (personnel, facilities, instruments), the process (the sequence of activities), the outcome (recipient health status or client satisfaction), the efficiency (the costs incurred to produce a certain outcome) and the effectiveness (frequency that the required results are attained). **Conclusion:** Careful attention must be paid to all aspects of the quality of donor tissues in order to maintain confidence in their safety and effectiveness. A well-managed QMS is a valuable and effective instrument to guarantee the required high standards for the donation, procurement, testing, processing, storage, distribution and traceability of ocular tissues as well as to facilitate the continuous improvement and the attainment of the objectives of an eye bank.

Introduction

The adoption and the correct operation of a *quality management system* (QMS) in an eye bank assures a high level of protection for the health of recipients of ocular tissues [1–10].

A *management system* is defined as a set of coordinated activities to guide and control a group of people or intermediaries, with specific responsibilities, powers and interrelationships with regard to quality.

Quality is the level at which a set of intrinsic characteristics of a service meet the requirements (implicit or explicit) or expectations of the interested parties.

A QMS comprises the organisational structure, the responsibilities, procedures, processes and the resources assigned to carry out the control of quality, including all the activities that directly or indirectly contribute to quality.

A QMS reference model is the ISO 9001:2000 standard [7] which allows for the development and implementation of a system for the purpose of:

- furnishing general operative instructions for all personnel;
- providing an instrument capable of measuring the effectiveness and efficiency of processes;
- singling out areas of improvement;
- supplying a service able to satisfy the implicit and explicit needs of the interested parties with regard to the services delivered;
- measuring and improving the performance of the interested parties.

General Requirements

The development of a QMS is guided by the following principles:

- orientation of the interested parties (organisations or persons who receive the services delivered by an eye bank) intended as donor families, procurement/retrieval sites, patients, doctors or transplantation centres, by an ever more precise definition of the requirements that explain the expectations and the requirements of the parties themselves; health and safety protection of those people involved in the operative activities;
- utilization of the human resources;
- approach of the processes for the delivery of the services;
- valorisation of the intended role of the QMS as an instrument for the management of a continuous improvement and for the attainment of the objectives of an eye bank;
- progressive vision of how to improve services in the perspective of an organisation oriented towards excellence;
- decisions based on factual information obtained from an analysis of data and documented information;
- ratification (or qualification in the case of equipment or environments), or the production of documented proof, capable of guaranteeing to a high degree of certainty that determined proceedings, equipment or environments will give rise to a product that conforms to specifications and to prearranged qualitative characteristics: a process is ratified in order to assess whether a system functions effectively compared to the intended use.

For the design and development of a QMS, it is necessary to:

- identify the processes;

- establish the interactions, the criteria and the methods necessary to assure the effective functioning and verification;
- distinguish the requirements of the technical and human resources;
- individualise the information necessary to support the operation;
- determine the actions required to attain the planned results and constant improvement;
- define the ways of measurement, monitoring, analysis and improvement.

In the identification phase, it is important to distinguish the different process types which constitute an integrated whole of a single system.

Directional processes comprise: the definition and diffusion of the policy and the objectives coherent with the mission and the vision of the eye bank; the adoption of the undertakings and actions to guarantee the availability of resources, the monitoring and the re-examination of the results.

Support processes include: management of the technical and infrastructural resources; management and development of the human resources, quality, system of health protection and staff safety and the protection of the environment.

Outsourcing processes regard those activities entrusted to organisations external to the eye bank.

Requirements Relating to Documentation

Structure

The planning and development of a QMS is to a large extent centred on the definition of the documental architecture with a view to:

- single out the laws, the technical norms, the guidelines and the reference standards for the procurement, processing, evaluation, storage and distribution of ocular tissues;
- determine the structure and the hierarchy of the documents [format, content and the codification criteria of the standard operating procedures (SOPs) and registration forms];
- define the form of management of the documentation (elaboration, verification, approval, distribution and registration/filing);
- assure the coherence and homogeneity, particularly over time, between the system of documentation and the detailed operational activities;
- guarantee organisational, managerial and operative standards, applicable to and shared with the whole organisation of the eye bank and with other relevant structures, for example external third parties entrusted to carry out processes outsourced by the eye bank;
- assure the traceability of tissues at every stage of the procurement, processing, evaluation and storage phases, up to the distribution of the tissue to the recipient or place of disposal, including the capacity to determine the donor and tissue

establishment or the production centre that receives, processes or conserves tissue and, at the level of medical structure, the ability to determine who was responsible for performing the transplantations to the tissue recipients; traceability also implies the capacity to trace and individualise all the pertinent information relating to products and materials that come into contact with each tissue.

Hence a document structure is divided as follows:

- laws, technical norms, guidelines and reference standards;
- eye bank authorisations and certifications;
- QMS manual;
- standard operative procedures;
- registration forms;
- documents for the planning, management and control of the process;
- monitoring and assessment of the activity.

The manual should include the:

- scope and the application field of the system;
- quality policy;
- legislative reference framework;
- eye bank's organisational set-up;
- design of the documentation system;
- description of the processes and their relative interactions with references to the SOPs.

SOPs are defined as written instructions that describe the phases of a determined process, as well as the materials and methods used and the final product expected.

Data, information and the results obtained in every phase of the procurement, processing, evaluation, storage and distribution of the tissues must be reported on the appropriate registration forms, in order to provide evidence of the activity undertaken, which constitute the fundamental instrument for assuring traceability.

Keeping under Control

The document structure and hierarchy (format, content and codification criteria of the SOPs and registration forms) and the form of management (elaboration, verification, approval, distribution, archiving) must be described in a detailed procedure.

In particular, the procedure should define the ways to:

a check and approve documents for adequacy prior to their use;
b re-examine and, when necessary, update and reapprove the same documents;
c identify the modifications and the state of the current revisions of the documents;
d ensure that the relevant versions of the applicable documents are available in the appropriate places of use;
e ensure that the documents are legible, and remain so, and that they are easily identifiable and retraceable;

f assure that documents which originate from outside come to be identified and their distribution supervised;
g avoid the involuntary use of out-of-date documents and chose a suitable archive identification if they are to be preserved (for legal reasons and/or conservation of the know-how).

Passage of Circulation

For every document there should be a defined corresponding course of circulation, generally articulated in the phases of drafting, authentication, approval and distribution. Prior to distribution the completeness and adequacy of the documents must be verified and approved by the person in charge of the eye bank.

Distribution

Documents are distributed to staff in a controlled manner. Confirmation of the consignment must be made by asking each staff member to sign the pertinent distribution registration form(s).

Modifications

Modifications are made in the event of:
- changes in the organisational structure;
- new legislative requirements, guidelines, statutes and/or regulations;
- new operative requirements;
- new medical-scientific knowledge;
- corrective and/or preventive interventions on the QMS;
- changes and/or the introduction of new processes.

Changes introduced to documents must be verified and approved by the person in charge of the eye bank so as to ensure the congruence between the introduced modifications and the original draft of the document.

Filing and Archive Keeping

The eye bank must plan suitable ways to:
- assure correct filing and document storage;
- guarantee suitable forms of access;
- avoid deterioration, damage or loss of documents and data, whether in paper, magnetic or optic format.

Paper and electronic archives must be organised in such a way as to ensure the protection and reference of the documents, as well as a secure conservation of the same for the decreed period.

Documentation bearing personal and/or sensitive information must be managed in accordance with the modalities laid down in the applicable personal data protection legislation.

Invalid and/or Out-of-Date Documents

Invalid and/or out-of-date documents must be promptly removed from all the emission/utilization points and appropriately identified with a notice (for example: 'inoperative') in order to avoid the inappropriate use of the same. The historical collection of QMS documentation must be conserved for a fixed period of time (30 years in the case of the Italian regulations).

Management of the Documents for the Registration of Quality

Records should provide evidence of compliance with the requisites of the QMS, and its efficient functioning, and should be organised and conserved so as to be legible, easily identifiable and traceable. Records are conserved for a fixed period of time (30 years for Italy) in order to provide evidence of the compliance with the requisites and of the efficient functioning of the QMS.

Resource Management

Available Resources

For the purpose of assuring the delivery of services in accordance with the established requisites and standards, the eye bank must determine and make available the necessary resources. Such resources must be suitable and related to the nature of the activity carried out, target-oriented to pursue the objectives established in the quality policy, and implement and maintain the QMS, so as to constantly improve its efficiency and effectiveness.

Human Resources

The personnel must be sufficient in number and qualified for the tasks carried out. The competence of each person must be periodically evaluated. Job descriptions must be clear, documented and updated. In addition, the relative tasks, competencies and responsibilities must be well documented and inclusive.

Initial basic training must be guaranteed to all staff, along with the necessary refresher courses when procedures change or when there is a development in scientific knowledge, as well as suitable equivalent professional development opportunities.

The programme of information, formation and vocational training must guarantee and document that each person has:

a shown competence in the carrying out of the expected tasks;
b demonstrated knowledge and adequate understanding of the processes and scientific/technical principles underpinning the intended tasks;
c understood the organisational framework, the quality system and the relevant health and safety standards in the field of eye and tissue banking;
d been adequately informed of the wider ethical, legislative and regulatory context of their own work.

A suitable procedure must be prepared in advance for the management of the human resources and in particular must contain:

- the competencies required for each role in relation to the tasks assigned and to the relative responsibilities;
- the procedures relative to the selection, evaluation and insertion of new staff members;
- the planning, programming and execution of the activity of information, formation and vocational staff training;
- the manner for verifying the efficacy of the information, formation and vocational staff training modules and periodic checks of staff competencies;
- the ways of recording and reporting the activity for the purpose of monitoring the support and the professional development of the human resources, also in relation to the duties and responsibilities assigned.

Infrastructure and Work Environment

Each eye bank must have suitable facilities to carry out their activity. The planning and the maintenance of all the equipment and materials must correspond to their expected purpose and minimise all potential risks for the intended recipients and/or medical personnel.

The infrastructure comprises: buildings, work spaces and connected facilities; eye bank equipment and instrumentation; support services.

All the equipment and critical technical apparatus must be identified and ratified, periodically inspected and subjected to preventive maintenance in compliance with the manufacturer's instructions.

Particular attention should also be paid to the working environment, intended as the totality of the conditions (physical, social, psychological and environmental factors) in which the activities are carried out and which constitute the basis for the functioning of the processes.

Special procedures must define the duties, responsibilities and the means for the:

- qualification of the equipment and the tissue-processing environments;
- management of the equipment and the technical apparatus;
- cleaning, cleansing and disinfection of the environments;
- management of biohazard waste;
- management of the infrastructure and the work environment as a whole (equipment etc.) in order to guarantee observance of the health and safety laws and to define the behaviour code in case of emergencies and/or incidents.

For the protection of the health and safety of staff, particular attention must be directed at:

- guaranteeing that all activities come to be carried out with the most rigorous respect for the safety regulations connected to the particular field of action(s);
- avoiding dangerous work situations, incidents, accidents and occupational diseases;
- continuously improving the health and safety conditions at work;
- managing those activities in an effective and efficient manner.

To this end, procedures must be put into practice and specific activities formalised for the:

- characterisation of the dangers;
- evaluation of the risks;
- determination of the prevention and protection measures;
- planning of the controls;
- monitoring and measurements necessary to guarantee the effectiveness of the system;
- management of emergencies;
- management of incidents and accidents;
- training and information of staff, suppliers and contractors;
- determination of the objectives for improvement;
- activation of improvement programmes.

Organisation and Management of the Processes

In general, the requirements of an organisational, managerial and technical-professional nature, relating to services and assistance offered by the bank, can arise from a number of different sources:

- requirements expressed by interested parties (patients, relatives, citizens/users, doctors etc.);
- conditions defined by the bank;
- compulsory requisites (legislative requirements);

- technical-professional provisions (guidelines, recommendations, scientific evidence);
- stipulations of a contractual nature (agreements with transplantation centres);
- implicit requisites of various interested parties.

Such requisites are substantiated in the requests from interested parties and registered in the apposite internal documents.

Prior to accepting a request for assistance, the bank has the responsibility to verify whether it is able to fully meet the expectations and requirements of the applicant.

The verification is intended to:

- guarantee the correct interpretation of the applicant's requirements and needs;
- check the technical, organisational and managerial capacity to deliver the assistance and services requested, in observance of the contractual stipulations (explicit and implicit);
- point out and resolve an eventual criticality which might compromise the effectiveness of the assistance and/or satisfaction of the client;
- resolve possible differences between the requirements requested and those previously formalised;
- point out responsibilities and reciprocal commitments;
- highlight possible forms of protection/security.

In front of eventual modifications to the specifications of the product/service, the bank must assure that the relevant contractual and informative documents are re-examined and that the staff concerned are made aware of these modifications.

Information relating to the assistance offered can be communicated for example in the following ways:

- service guides;
- informative material distributed inside the bank;
- informative material distributed to interested parties;
- phone contacts, web site (if present).

The eye bank must undertake a protective role towards the interested parties, even considering the possibility of complaints following bad service or a non-conformity/adverse reaction/event.

Tissue Procurement

The retrieval of human tissues should be undertaken by personnel who have successfully completed a specific training programme. The eye bank establishes the procedures to follow in order to assure conformity to the donor selection criteria, the proper enucleation and excision techniques and the reconstruction of the donor body.

SOPs must be defined in order to verify the:

a identity of the donor;
b documentation relating to the consent to donate given by the family;

c appraisal of the donor selection criteria;
d evaluation of the laboratory tests requested for the donors.

Furthermore SOPs must be defined for the retrieval, packaging, labelling and transport of tissue to the eye bank.

Tissue retrieval must take place in suitably assessed facilities, following the correct aseptic techniques, in order to minimise bacterial and other types of contamination of the tissues during procurement.

Materials and equipment used for retrieval should be properly supervised, taking into account the regulations and norms, and applicable national and international guidelines, relating to the sterilisation of medicinal and medical devices. For tissue retrievals, qualified sterile instruments and devices (preferably single-use) must be employed.

A unique identification code must be assigned to the donor, as well as each individual donated tissue, either by the tissue procurement organisation or by the receiving bank, so as to guarantee a satisfactory identification of the donor and the traceability of the donated tissues.

Documentation relating to the donor should be conserved in a way that puts into practice data protection and safeguard measures in order to avoid unauthorised data additions, suppressions or modifications. There must be no unauthorised disclosure of information, guaranteeing at the same time the retraceability of the donations and ensuring that the identity of the recipient(s) is not revealed to the donor's family or vice versa.

Tissue Reception

When retrieved tissues arrive at the eye bank, it is necessary to carry out a documented check of the condition of the shipment, the packaging, the labelling as well as the documentation and any enclosed blood samples.

Tissues and receipts must be kept in quarantine until such materials and their pertinent documentation have been examined or otherwise controlled. If not previously done, a unique identification code must be attributed to the donor and donated tissues. The examination of the information relating to the donor and retrieval, as well as the resulting acceptance of the donor, must be performed by suitably trained and authorised personnel.

Tissue Processing

The critical processing procedures must be ratified and must not render the tissues clinically ineffective or noxious to the recipient. Such validations can be based on studies carried out by the bank, on data from published studies or – for processing procedures which are well known – on retrospective evaluation of clinical results relating to tissues furnished by the bank.

Procedures must be documented in the SOPs and must guarantee that all the processes are carried out in conformity with the approved SOPs.

Before each significant processing modification, the modified process must be ratified and documented.

The processing procedures must periodically be subjected to critical analysis in order to assure that they continue to attain the intended results.

Procedures to discard tissues must prevent the contamination of other tissues, the working environment and staff. Such procedures must follow national regulations.

Storage and Declaration of Tissue Suitability

A maximum duration must be specified for each type of storage condition. The time chosen must take account of the probable deterioration of the characteristics of the tissues.

A control system is needed to guarantee that tissues are not declared suitable before all the selection procedures have been respected: the bank must thus equip itself with a SOP which specifies the circumstances, the responsibilities and the procedures applicable to the release of tissues for distribution.

The system for the identification of tissues in every phase of processing must clearly differentiate between those in quarantine and those discarded. Records must show that all the corresponding conditions have been observed prior to tissue release: in particular that all the declaration forms in use, the relevant medical records, the processing records and the testing results have been verified according to a written procedure by an operator authorised for this purpose by the person in charge of the bank. If a telematic system is used to communicate laboratory testing results, a control trace must indicate the person responsible for declaring tissue suitability.

It is necessary to undertake a documented estimation of the risks, approved by the person in charge of the bank, to decide the fate of all stored tissues after the introduction of new criteria for the selection or screening of donors or notable modifications to the processing phases, with the object of reinforcing safety and/or quality.

Distribution and Recall

The bank is required to define the critical conditions for tissue transport, such as temperature and expiry date, in order to maintain the requested properties of the tissues.

The container/packaging must be secure and guarantee the preservation of the tissues in the conditions specified. All the containers and packaging must be ratified as suitable for the purpose.

If the distribution is entrusted to a third party, it in necessary to have a documented agreement which guarantees the maintenance of the requested conditions.

In addition, there is a need to have an effective recall procedure, which should include a description of the responsibilities and the actions to undertake, including the notification of the competent authorities. Actions must be embarked upon within a predefined period, provide for the traceability of the tissues concerned and, if required, include a reconstruction of events. Investigations should aim to identify each donor who may have contributed to or caused a reaction in a recipient, to recuperate the tissues originating from such a donor and to inform recipients (or intended recipients) of tissues retrieved from that donor of the potential risk to which they could be exposed to.

The bank must prepare in advance procedures for the handling of tissue requests. Procedures for the allocation of tissues to determined patients or transplantation centres must be documented and communicated at their request.

It is also necessary to have a documented system for the handling of returned tissues, comprising, if need be, the criteria for their entry in the register.

Equipment and Materials

The planning and maintenance of all the equipment and materials must correspond to their expected purposes and minimise every risk for the potential recipients and/or staff.

All the equipment and critical technical apparatus must be identified and ratified, periodically inspected and subjected to preventive maintenance in compliance with the manufacturer's instructions. The equipment or materials which affect critical parameters of processing or storage (for example temperature, pressure, particle counts and levels of microbial contamination) must be identified and if necessary subjected to examination, supervision, alarms and suitable corrective interventions to determine any dysfunctions and defects in order to guarantee that the critical parameters constantly remain below the acceptable limits. All the equipment that has a critical measuring function must be calibrated according to an available reference standard, if one exists.

New or repaired equipment must be checked at the moment of installation and validated prior to use. The results of the controls must be documented.

Procedures must allow for the periodic maintenance, cleaning and disinfection of all the critical equipment and the resulting registration of such activities.

The operating norms for each piece of critical apparatus must be clearly displayed, with detailed instructions of how to intervene in case of malfunction or breakdown.

The standards for the activity in which accreditation/designation/authorisation/licensing is sought must indicate in detail the specifications of all the critical materials and reagents. In particular the analytical descriptions for the additions (e.g. solutions) and the packaging materials must be defined. The reagents and critical materials must correspond to the legal regulations and to documented provisions and, if applicable, to the prescriptions of European Directive 93/42/CEE of 14 June 1993 [4] concerning medical devices and Directive 98/79/EC [5] of the European Parliament and of the Council of 27 October 1998 regarding in vitro diagnostic medical devices.

Monitoring and Measuring

Measurements, Analyses and Improvement

The bank should have, within the scope of their QMS, plans and actual processes for monitoring, measuring, analysing and introducing improvements necessary to:

- demonstrate conformity of the services delivered and assistance given;
- assure the consistency of the QMS;
- develop in a continuous fashion the efficiency of the QMS.

The bank should establish a feedback system specifically designed to monitor information regarding:

- its capacity to identify the needs of its clients and the supply of services which it is capable of satisfying;
- the perception of its clients on how far the organisation has satisfied the determined and expected requisites.

For an analysis of client satisfaction, prepared suitable evaluation questionnaires are administered to patients and collaborating transplant surgeons. The returned data are analysed and converted into statistical form in order to reveal the level of satisfaction, as perceived by the interested parties, and to define any targeted action, if any, required to improve the quality of the delivered services and assistance offered. The results of this analysis should be discussed and examined.

Internal Audits

The procedure for the QMS must define the manner in which internal audits are managed for the purpose of verifying the efficiency and the coherence of the eye bank's QMS.

The procedure should set out:

- the criteria, extent and periodicity of the controls;
- the tasks and requisites for planning the inspections;
- the responsibilities and modalities for documenting the results of the internal audits and the conservation of the relating records;
- the responsibility for those actions necessary to eradicate the exposed non-compliances and their causes.

The audits should:

- be planned and systematic in accordance with the cadence of the agreed programme;
- be carried out in conformity with operative instructions based on written procedures;
- be conducted on the basis of a list of predefined controls (checklist);
- give rise to facts (or data) by which a judgement can be made, based on objective evidence;
- take into consideration the conformity to the procedures, the regulations, the instructions and specifications that constitute the regulative and realised structure of the audited QMS;
- document the results.

The audits must be conducted by persons who are independent from those who have direct responsibility for the activity undergoing the audit.

Monitoring and Measuring of the Processes

The QMS must adopt adequate methods to monitor and measure the processes, in order to verify the capacity of the processes to obtain the planned results. If such results are not attained, corrections must be adopted and corrective actions undertaken to assure conformity of the services.

The indicators of measure are fixed for the primary processes and data discussed during the review by the management.

Monitoring and Measuring of the Services

The QMS must adopt adequate methods to monitor and measure the performance of the services delivered and to verify that the relative requisites have been satisfied. The monitoring and measurement activities should also be carried out in all the subprocesses.

Evidence of the conformity to the approved criteria should be documented in the appropriate records. These should also indicate the person(s) who is authorised to issue/release a product or service. The release of a product and delivery of a service must not be carried out prior to the successful completion of the foreseen controls.

Management of Non-Conformities

The management of the non-conformities should set out the ways to handle all non-compliances revealed by or to the eye bank staff during the execution of their activities so as to guarantee that:

- those performances and processes that do not conform are identified, managed, recorded and kept under control, with particular reference to adverse reactions or events correlated with the use of tissues revealed as a result of process reviews or communications from transplantation centres;
- services or process results that do not comply with the relevant requirements are identified and kept under control to avoid their involuntary use or dispatch, or used as a consequence of particular situations or according to precise conditions;
- those elements of the quality system that do not conform are promptly pointed out so that they can be brought back to a level of acceptability.

The person in charge of the bank must establish the necessary operative procedures to adopt appropriate preventive or corrective actions with respect to actual or probable effects consequential to potential or ascertained non-compliances of the processes or services delivered.

Data Analysis

The eye bank analyses data for the purpose of obtaining information with regard to:

- client satisfaction;
- conformity to the service requirements;
- the features of the progress/advancement of the processes and services;
- the performance of the suppliers.

Statistical reports containing data and information relative to the activities undertaken should be elaborated on a periodic basis. Such reports should be distributed to all delegated personnel and discussed during the course of internal informative meetings.

Continuous Improvement

The bank continuously ameliorates the efficiency of the quality system, using the results from the survey of client satisfaction and data that emerges from the statistical reports.

Improvements to the system should be decided during the management review phase and the period for executing and ratifying the efficiency established.

Corrective Actions

Corrective actions are defined as 'actions undertaken to eliminate the causes of a non-conformity, defects in existence or other undesirable situations, in order to avoid them being repeated'.

They are considered as being fundamental instruments to act upon the causes of the non-conformities with a view to avoiding that these become repetitive.

The activation of a corrective action can be requested as a consequence of a submitted report and/or communication from an informative source, such as:

- non compliance reports;
- reclaims;
- audit reports.

It is important to point out that corrective actions are not intended to correct a non-conformity (in which case one talks of a correction or handling of the non-conformity), but rather to intervene in the cause which has generated the non-conformity, so as to avoid a repetition of the same.

Following the revelation of a non-conformity, the relevant causes must be analysed and a decision made by the person in charge of the bank as to whether a corrective action needs to be embarked upon. In the event that it is considered necessary, the opening of a corrective action must be made on the appropriate form, and the time needed to carry out the corrective action, the person responsible and actions to perform clearly articulated.

Periodically the person in charge of the bank and the quality manager must verify the effectiveness of the corrective actions put into practice.

Preventive Actions

Preventive actions are defined as 'actions taken to eliminate the causes of potential non-conformities or other potential undesirable situations'.

The sources for the activation of a preventive action are represented in general by:

- audit reports;
- results arising from an analysis of statistical data;
- results from a monitoring of the process indicators;
- modifications to the legislative reference framework;
- analysis of client satisfaction;
- benchmarking.

Every preventive action is characterised by a life cycle which is articulated in the following phases:

- identification of the potential non-conformity and/or area of improvement;
- determination of the possible causes of the non-conformity;
- determination of the necessary preventive actions;
- putting into practice the preventive actions;
- registration of the results of the actions undertaken;
- re-examination of the adopted preventive actions (verifying the effectiveness of the actions adopted).

A preventive action can be defined from whatever organisational position that may involve an area of potential non-conformity and/or improvement. Preventive actions should be discussed and reviewed by the management for verification of their execution and effectiveness.

References

1 Directive 2004/23/EC of the European Parliament and of the Council of 31 March 2004 on setting standards of quality and safety for the donation, procurement, testing, processing, preservation, storage and distribution of human tissues and cells. Official Journal of the European Union, L 102/48, 7 April 2004.

2 Commission Directive 2006/17/EC of 8 February 2006 implementing Directive 2004/23/EC of the European Parliament and of the Council as regards certain technical requirements for the donation, procurement and testing of human tissues and cells. Official Journal of the European Union, L 38/40, 9 February 2006.

3 Commission Directive 2006/86/EC of 24 October 2006 implementing Directive 2004/23/EC of the European Parliament and of the Council as regards traceability requirements, notification of serious adverse reactions and events and certain technical requirements for the coding, processing, preservation, storage and distribution of human tissues and cells. Official Journal of the European Union, L 294/32, 25 October 2006.

4 Council Directive 93/42/EEC of 14 June 1993 concerning medical devices. Official Journal of the European Union, L 169, 12 July 1993, pp 1–43.

5 Directive 98/79/EC of the European Parliament and of the Council of 27 October 1998 on in vitro diagnostic medical devices. Official Journal of the European Union, L 331, 7 December 1998, pp 1–37.

6 European Council: Guide to safety and quality assurance for the transplantation of organs, tissues and cells – 3rd edition. Strasbourg, Council of Europe, 2007.

7 International Organization for Standardization: Quality management systems – requirements (EN ISO 9001:2000). Geneva, International Organization for Standardization, December 2000.

8 International Organization for Standardization: Quality management systems – fundamentals and vocabulary (EN ISO 9000:2000). Geneva, International Organization for Standardization, December 2000.

9 International Organization for Standardization: Quality management systems – guidelines for performance improvements (EN ISO 9004:2000). Geneva, International Organization for Standardization, December 2000.

10 International Organization for Standardization: Guidelines for quality and/or environmental management systems auditing (EN ISO 19011:2002). Geneva, International Organization for Standardization, October 2002.

Mauro Toniolo
Quality Manager
Fondazione Banca degli Occhi del Veneto – ONLUS
Via Paccagnella n. 11 – Padiglione Rama
IT–30174 Zelarino – Venice (Italy)
Tel. +39 041 9656446, Fax +39 041 9656401, E-Mail mauro.toniolo@fbov.it

Bredehorn-Mayr T, Duncker GIW, Armitage WJ (eds): Eye Banking.
Dev Ophthalmol. Basel, Karger, 2009, vol 43, pp 87–96

Allocation of Corneas in Europe

Arlinke G. Bokhorst · Caroline A. Dorrepaal

BIS Foundation, Leiden, The Netherlands

Abstract

Background: To safeguard a fair distribution of available corneas, (inter)national and regional allocation principles have to be developed and implemented. **Methods:** To obtain information about allocation principles over the world, a literature search was done. Allocation in Europe was investigated by international data of Bio Implant Services Foundation (BIS) over the period 2002–2007. **Results:** For 4 different types of corneal grafts, e.g. random, HLA-typed, lamellar and emergency corneas, different allocation principles are described. Applying allocation criteria leads to dynamics in the donor and patient pool, which could be monitored by establishing the mean waiting time for each kind of corneal graft. Specific attention should be given to the division of corneas over the pools of different graft types, to ensure equal access to a transplant for all cornea patients. **Conclusions:** Due to new surgical techniques and seasonal changes in the supply of corneal grafts, allocation is a dynamic process, which has to be closely monitored.

Necessity to Regulate Cornea Allocation

The need to set rules for allocation of corneas to keratoplasty patients is principally based on the Convention on Human Rights and Biomedicine, which declares that member states of the European Council should take measures to assure 'an equitable access to healthcare of appropriate quality' for all its inhabitants [1]. The main incentive to regulate the access to cornea transplants occurs when the supply of corneas does not meet the clinical demand. This could be permanently the case, but since corneas have a limited shelf life, there can easily arise periods in which the demand for corneas outnumbers the available corneas in the bank or vice versa. Beside the absolute availability of corneas, another important reason for managing the allocation of corneas is to be able to match HLA genotypes of corneal grafts with potential recipients.

When patients are forced to wait for a corneal graft and waiting lists arise, some kind of prioritizing has to be developed. According to the guiding principles of the WHO for allocation of organs, tissues and cells, these rules should be guided by clinical and ethical norms, without any other (financial) considerations. Moreover, these rules should be equitable, externally justified, transparent and defined by constituted bodies consisting of experts in the field of medicine, bioethics and public health (guiding principle 9) [2]. Depending on the healthcare structure and the volume of patients, these allocation rules can be applied on local, regional and/or (inter) national levels.

Allocation Principles

Several criteria can be used to prioritize the patients who are in need of a cornea transplant. In general, the principles for allocation should be based on medical indication, urgency and prospects of success. Unethical aspects such as gender, race and financial capacity of the recipient or surgical center must be rejected as factor of importance in the ranking of patients [3].

The following aspects could be eligible as principles for allocation of corneas.

Medical Aspects

- Underlying cornea disease (factors like pain, rapid progression, prognosis without transplant)
- Chance of graft rejection (previous rejections, immunological risk factors)
- Clinical urgency to save the function of the eye (e.g. perforation)
- Correspondence between donor and recipient age

Social Aspects

- Time spent on the waiting list
- National or regional balance between number of donations and transplantations
- Ability to cope with visual dysfunction
- Social consequences of blindness

Which criteria should be taken into account and with what weight factor, will be determined by the local balance in demand and supply and the importance that society attaches to the above-mentioned medical and social aspects. The purpose of an allocation algorithm is to provide a society-based and fair division of the available corneas, to safeguard the equal access of patients to donated corneas and to guarantee that patients are treated in the order of their medical urgency (provided that transplantation improves their condition). Special care should be given to the availability of corneas for patients who are in urgent need of a transplant (<5 days) to safeguard the function of the eye.

Table 1. Country of origin of donors and recipients of corneas allocated through BIS Foundation in the period from January 1, 2002, to December 31, 2007

Origin of patients	Origin of cornea		Total
	The Netherlands	Other European countries	
Great Britain	1	0	1
Norway	1	0	1
The Netherlands	4,484	177	4,661
Belgium	59	15	74
Germany	2,774	441	3,215
Austria	57	10	67
Switzerland	18	2	20
Italy	121	17	138
Greece	216	6	222
Israel	10		10
Tunisia	14		14
Libya	8		8
Total	7,763	668	8,431

The Organization of Cornea Allocation in the Netherlands in an International Context

In the Netherlands a national system of cornea donation and allocation exists. Potential cornea donors are reported to a central call center, which is operated by BIS Foundation. After initial medical screening, BIS Foundation organizes the procurement and transportation of the bulbi to the cornea banks. The cornea bank assesses the quality of the corneas and reports this information back to BIS Foundation. BIS Foundation keeps a constant overview of the available corneas.

In the meantime, Dutch patients in need of corneas are reported to BIS Foundation and registered on a waiting list. To optimize demand and supply, patients from other European countries are registered on the waiting list as well. Moreover, BIS Foundation collaborates with several cornea banks in Europe to be able to supply to all the patients on the waiting list. By means of this network the pool of (potentially) available corneas can be enlarged, which will improve the chance of patients to receive the most suitable cornea (like for HLA-matched corneas) or meet temporal discrepancies in local demand and supply. Table 1 shows the international exchange of corneas. Over the period 2002–2007, 8,431 corneas were exchanged through this network of international collaboration. Of these, 55% (n = 4,661) was allocated to Dutch patients. The remaining 45% (n = 3,770) was distributed to patients from 8 different European countries and 3 countries outside Europe. The majority (65%)

of corneas is transplanted as at random cornea in a perforating keratoplasty (among which 6% are emergency procedures), 28% was allocated as HLA-matched cornea and 7% was used for lamellar applications.

At BIS Foundation the available corneas are allocated to patients on the waiting list, according to a set of allocation rules [4], which are designed and approved by an international committee of experts in the field of cornea transplantation. When it concerns corneas donated by Dutch donors, the allocation criteria are furthermore approved by the Dutch Transplant Foundation, which is a semi-governmental organization.

Dynamics of Cornea Allocation

Depending on the type of corneal graft, different kinds of medical and social factors play a role in the prioritizing process. Therefore each type of corneal graft allocation has its own dynamics and needs to be organized and controlled in a different way. The following types of allocation of corneal grafts can be recognized:

- allocation of random corneas;
- allocation of random corneas for emergency treatment;
- allocation of HLA-matched corneas;
- allocation of corneas for lamellar transplantation.

To ensure equal access to corneas for all patients, not only allocation algorithms have to be developed per type of corneal graft, but also rules to make sure that the availability of corneas is fairly distributed among the above-mentioned groups.

Characteristics of Random Allocation of Corneas Including Emergency Situations

In general the allocation of random corneas is characterized by two factors: the degree of shortage and the relative limited shelf life of corneas. When shortage is experienced, medical conditions, like pre-existing diseases and waiting time are the most likely tools to prioritize patients for transplantation.

A special situation occurs when transplantation has to take place within hours to days, like in case of a threatening perforation. According to allocation criteria, BIS Foundation gives these urgent patients priority over those waiting for more elective surgery. When corneas are preserved in organ culture, deswelling and culturing of these corneas may take 2–3 days. To ensure sufficient corneas for immediate use, special provisions have to be made. Either a pool of 'ready for use' corneas has to be kept for those situations, or a cornea, which is already prepared for transplantation, has to be reallocated, and the planned operation has to be cancelled [5]. Since it is always hard to predict how many emergency corneas have to be stored in order to provide for these situations without wasting too many corneas when there is no demand, this type of allocation lends itself pre-eminently for (inter)national cooperation and exchange.

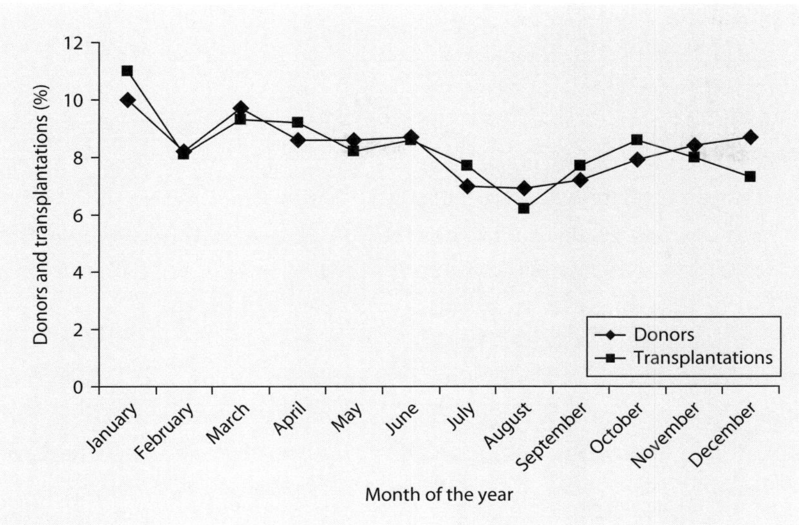

Fig. 1. Distribution of donations and transplantations through the year in the period from January 1, 2002, to December 31, 2007.

To optimize the outcome of transplantation in younger patients, BIS Foundation uses a maximum age difference between donor and patient of 30 years. Younger patients are expected to be retransplanted several times in their lifetime. To make the transplant last longer, high-quality endothelium is required, which is more often seen in younger donors [6, 7]. For pediatric patients this is especially hard to achieve, since in the BIS population there are more than 3 times as much patients as donors under the age of 18 years (1.7 vs. 0.5%). BIS Foundation has solved this problem by prioritizing pediatric patients above all other patient groups, when a cornea from a younger deceased donor becomes available.

When the supply of corneas is more or less in balance with the demand, the limited shelf life of corneas (organ culture ±4 weeks, cold storage 7–10 days) [8] still requires some management of allocation, in order to prevent wastages due to expiration. Furthermore, discrepancies between the availability of donors and operating capacity of hospitals and surgeons make coordination and tuning necessary, especially since donation and transplantation of corneas fluctuate over the year (fig. 1).

Complexity of HLA-Matched Cornea Allocation

After the discovery that immune reactions to HLA class I as well as HLA class II play a role in corneal graft rejection, studies have been developed to investigate the effect of HLA matching. The beneficial effect of HLA-A, -B and -DR matching has been shown in several studies [9, 10]. Not only in patients who have a high risk for graft failure due to immunological risk factors, but also in those with a normal risk profile has HLA matching been shown to improve graft survival [11]. Nevertheless, HLA matching is not generally applied. The main reason for this is that the improvement in graft survival has to be weighed against the additional time on the waiting list to find an HLA-suitable donor [12]. Although a prediction model has been developed [13] (and is currently validated by our own group) to estimate the time on the waiting list for an HLA-typed corneal graft, it is not possible to predict exactly when a suitable matched cornea will become available. Therefore the operation of HLA-matched corneal grafts cannot be scheduled like random cornea keratoplasties.

The chance of finding a fully matched cornea in a donor population depends on the percentage of donors with the same HLA typing and varies from 1.46% of potentially suitable donors for common HLA genotypes to approximately zero for rare typings. To optimize the chance of finding a suitable donor, the pool of HLA-typed corneas has to be as large as possible. International collaboration, whereby all available HLA corneas are centrally matched to an international waiting list of recipients registered for an HLA-typed cornea, is the only way to enhance the chance to find an HLA-suitable cornea within an acceptable waiting time for each patient. To achieve this, the Netherlands collaborates with German [14], Italian and Belgian cornea banks to exchange HLA-typed corneas. Together this collaboration forms the largest pool of HLA corneas in the world. Figure 2 shows the origin and number of HLA-typed patients that have been registered at BIS Foundation over the last 10 years.

Special care should be given to the availability of corneas for patients who are in urgent need of a transplant (<5 days) to safeguard the function of the eye.

HLA matching at BIS Foundation is performed by a computerized ranking algorithm. Patients are ranked for a given HLA-typed cornea according to the number of mismatches on broad HLA type I and II antigens. When 2 or more patients have a equal number of mismatches, the highest position on the ranking list will be given to patients with urgency factors like homozygosity on the A, B or DR locus, high antibody profile (panel-reactive antibody >5%) or previous graft rejection. When still equally ranked, the patients are subsequently matched on HLA split level whereby the lowest number of mismatches prevails. Finally time spent on the waiting list determines the position on the ranking list. Figure 3 shows that the majority of patients that are transplanted through this allocation algorithm have waited less than 6 months for their HLA-matched cornea. Not all of these patients did receive a corneal graft with 0 HLA mismatches. Depending on medical and social aspects, treating surgeons considered 1 or 2 mismatches also acceptable for their patients, and in that way reduced the waiting time.

Lamellar Corneal Grafts and Consistency with Allocation of Other Cornea Types

Due to recent advances in surgical techniques, selective replacement of part of the cornea became a promising alternative to conventional penetrating keratoplasty [15].

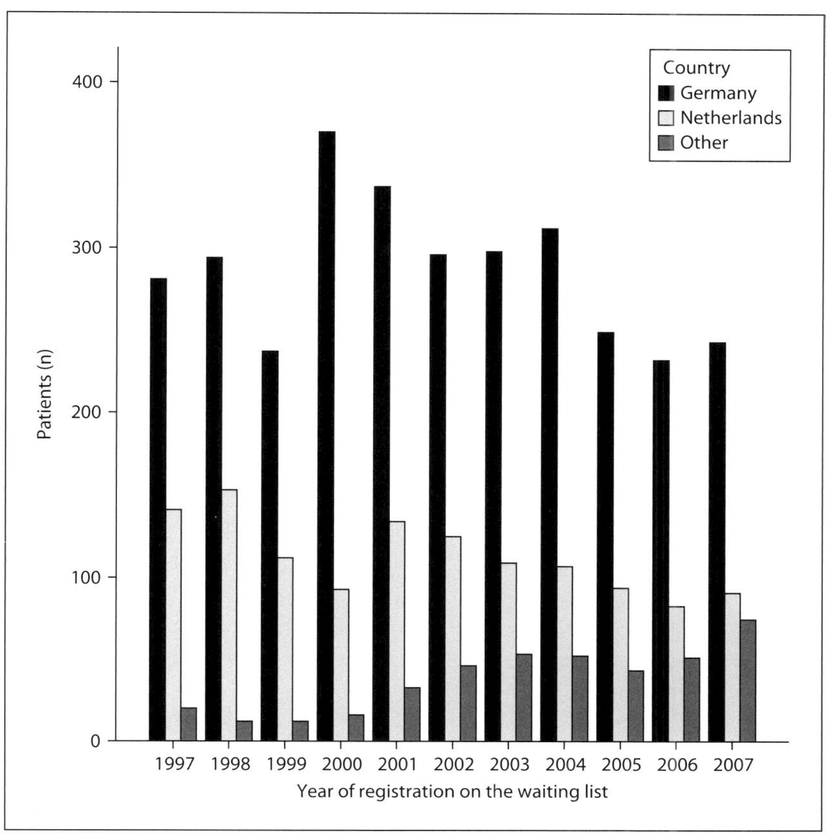

Fig. 2. Number of patients put on the waiting list for an HLA-typed corneal graft per country in the period from January 1, 2002, to December 31, 2007.

Preparation of anterior or posterior cornea layers is facilitated by devices such as automated microkeratome and Excimer laser and led to an increase in requests for lamellar grafts in the last few years as can be seen in figure 4. At the same time the number of patients registered for penetrating grafts decreased.

Initially the preparation of lamellar grafts was predominantly performed by the eye surgeons in the operating theater, but cornea banks are now taking over some of these preparations [16]. This makes allocation of lamellar corneas extra challenging, since corneas for these preparations have to be relatively fresh and therefore have to be allocated earlier in the process, than other types of corneal grafts.

Although patients are registered for different types of corneal grafts, often with different selection criteria, they have in principle an equal right to receive a graft. Since the lamellar selection criteria allow a cornea bank to accept small defects in the endothelium (anterior lamellar graft) or epithelial scars (posterior lamellar keratoplasty), the pool of corneas to allocate from differs from that of penetrating

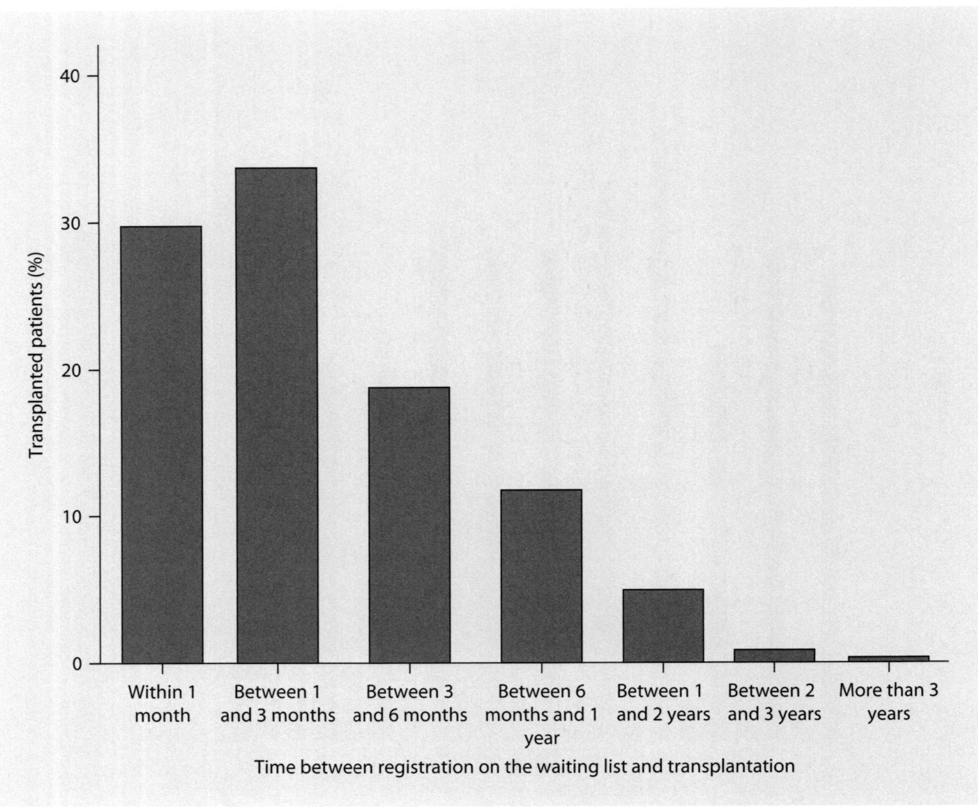

Fig. 3. Mean time between registration on the waiting list for an HLA-typed corneal graft and transplantation in the period from January 1, 2002, to December 31, 2007.

keratoplasty. By monitoring the average waiting time for the different types of corneal grafts and adjustment of allocation algorithms if necessary, equal access to the different types of keratoplasties can be safeguarded. In practice it means that the pool of lamellar corneas has to be enlarged with corneas suitable for perforating keratoplasty, when the waiting time for lamellar grafts becomes longer than that for a perforating keratoplasty. The same accounts for the number of HLA-typed versus random corneas. The balance between the number of corneas that are HLA-typed (and used as such) and the number of corneas left for at random keratoplasty has to be constantly monitored. If waiting times exceed certain preset levels, adjustments to the ratio of corneas in the different pools should be made.

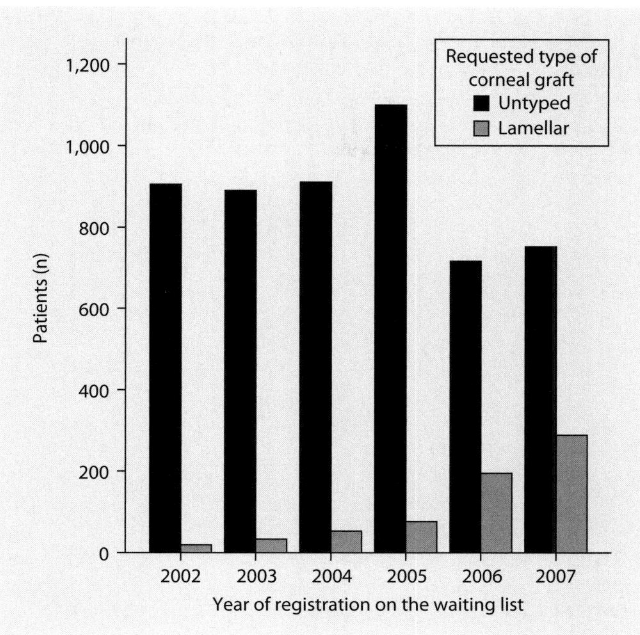

Fig. 4. Number of patients put on the waiting list for a lamellar or untyped corneal graft in the period from January 1, 2002, to December 31, 2007.

References

1 Council of Europe: Convention for the protection of human rights and dignity of the human being with regard to the application of biology and medicine: convention on human rights and biomedicine. ETS No 164. Strasbourg, Council of Europe, 1997.

2 WHO: Guiding principles on human tissue, cell and organ transplantation. Geneva, WHO, 2008.

3 World Medical Association: Statement on human organ and tissue donation and transplantation. Edinburgh, World Medical Association, 2000.

4 BIS allocation criteria: cornea. www.bisfoundation.org/allocation process.

5 Bredehorn T, Langer C, Duncker GIW, Wilhelm F: Constant availability of emergency cornea transplants in central German Corneabank Halle. Transplant Proc 2002;34:2351–2352.

6 Niederer RL, Perumal D, Sherwin T, McGhee CN: Age-related differences in the normal human cornea: a laser scanning in vivo confocal microscopy study. Br J Ophthalmol 2007;91:1165–1169.

7 Yee RW, Matsuda M, Schuktz RO, et al: Changes in the normal corneal endothelial cellular pattern as a function of age. Curr Eye Res 1985;4:671–678.

8 Pels E, Beele H, Claerhout I: Eye bank issues. II. Preservation techniques: warm versus cold storage. Int Ophthalmol 2008;28:155–163.

9 Volker-Dieben HJ, Claas FH, Schreuders FM, et al: Beneficial effect of HLA-DR matching on the survival of corneal allografts. Transplantation 2000;70: 640–648.

10 Khaireddin R, Wachtlin J, Hopfenmüller W, et al: HLA A, HLA B and HLA DR matching reduces the rate of corneal allograft rejection. Graefe's Arch Clin Exp Ophthalmol 2003;241:1020–1028.

11 Reinhard T, Boehringer D, et al: Improvement of graft prognosis in penetrating normal-risk keratoplasty by HLA class I and II matching. Eye 2004; 18:269–277.

12 Coster DJ, Williams KA: The impact of corneal allograft rejection on the long-term outcome of corneal transplantation. Am J Ophthalmol 2005;140: 1112–1122.

13 Böhringer D, Reinhard T, Böhringer S, et al: Predicting time on the waiting list for HLA matched corneal grafts. Tissue Antigens 2002;59:407–411.

14 Wissenschaftlicher Beirat der Bundesärztekammer: Richtlinien zum Führen einer Hornhautbank. August 7, 2000.

15 Tan DT, Mehta JS: Future directions in lamellar corneal transplantation. Cornea 2007;26(suppl 1):S21–S28.

16 Terry MA: Endothelial keratoplasty (EK): history, current state, and future directions. Cornea 2006; 25:873–878.

A.G. Bokhorst, Medical Director
BIS Foundation
PO Box 2304
NL–2301 CH Leiden (The Netherlands)
Tel. +31 71 5795840, Fax +31 71 5790903, E-Mail a.bokhorst@bisfoundation.nl

Bredehorn-Mayr T, Duncker GIW, Armitage WJ (eds): Eye Banking.
Dev Ophthalmol. Basel, Karger, 2009, vol 43, pp 97–104

Preparation and Preservation of Amniotic Membrane

Iva Dekaris · Nikica Gabrić

Eye Clinic 'Svjetlost', Zagreb, Croatia

Abstract

The human amniotic membrane (AM) is the innermost layer of the placenta and consists of a single epithelial layer, a thick basement membrane and an avascular stroma. Due to the number of its properties, AM is increasingly used in the treatment of severe ocular surface diseases. The amniotic basement membrane facilitates migration and growth of epithelial cells, therefore promoting epithelialization. The avascular stroma of the AM reduces fibrovascular ingrowth and abnormal neovascularization. Amniotic epithelium produces anti-inflammatory and growth factors beneficial to the treatment of inflammatory corneal diseases. AM is prepared from a fresh placenta under sterile conditions, washed with balanced salt solution containing penicillin, streptomycin, neomycin and amphotericin B, placed in tissue culture and glycerol at a ratio of 1:1, and stored at –80°C. A donor serological test for human immunodeficiency virus and hepatitis B and C viruses has to be all negative. After transplantation of the amniotic membrane (AMT) onto the eye surface, AM will be slowly absorbed within approximately 4–6 weeks. Depending on consumption, amniotic membranes are used up to 1 year after preparation, although many have recommended storage for an indefinite period. Since AM is not a completely transparent tissue, the patient's visual acuity may decrease after AMT; the patient should be aware of this temporary effect prior to surgery.

Amniotic Membrane Preparation

Amniotic membrane (AM) is obtained under sterile conditions from a human placenta obtained shortly after elective caesarean delivery. Informed consent is obtained from each donor, and screening is made to exclude any risk of transmissible infections such as human immunodeficiency virus, hepatitis virus types B and C, and syphilis. The placenta is first washed free of blood clots with balanced saline solution containing 50 μg/ml of penicillin, 50 μg/ml of streptomycin, 100 μg/ml of neomycin and 2.5 μg/ml of amphotericin B. Then the AM is separated from the rest of the chorion and rinsed with the balanced saline solution containing antibiotics. Under a laminar flow

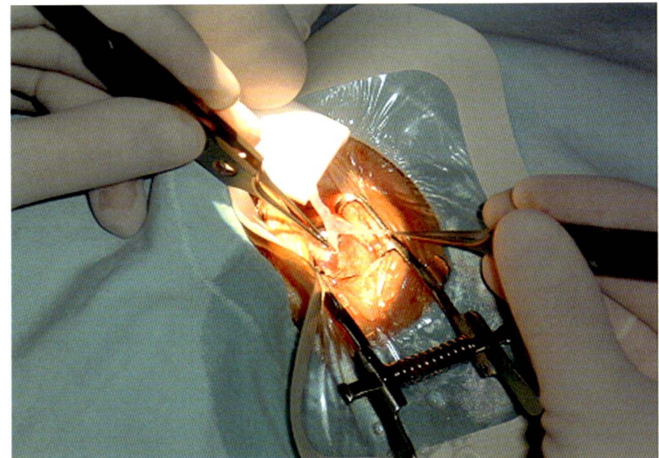

Fig. 1. Amniotic membrane transplantation. During surgery, AM is peeled off the nitrocellulose paper and cut to cover the ocular surface, with the epithelial surface facing up.

hood, the AM is cut into required sizes (most often 3 cm × 4 cm pieces, but other dimensions are also available) and flattened onto individually sterilized nitrocellulose paper without folds or tears with the epithelial surface up. Each AM is placed in a sterile vial containing tissue culture (e.g. Corneamax) and glycerol at a ratio of 1:1, and stored at –80°C. Depending on consumption, AM is used up to 1 year after preparation, although many have recommended storage for an indefinite period. Before use in the operating theatre, AM is thawed by leaving the vial at room temperature, and then the membrane is transferred to the ocular surface (fig. 1).

The AM may also be cryopreserved or freeze-dried, and as such it can last for a couple of years (mostly used in the USA). If the freeze-dried AM is used, care should be taken to rehydrate it properly before its clinical use. The time suggested for rehydration may vary from one supplier to another; the user should follow the instructions coming with the tissue. Although cryopreserved AM also has beneficial effects in the treatment of ocular surface diseases, it is still unclear whether beneficial anti-inflammatory and growth factors can survive cryopreservation.

Indications for Amniotic Membrane Transplantation

Several ocular surface disturbances caused by physical or chemical injuries, infections or systemic disorders may cause scarring of the conjunctiva or result in persistent ocular inflammation, primarily or secondarily involving the cornea. If severe, disturbances of the ocular surface may lead to significant visual impairment. Treatment of such a patient is challenging, often unsatisfactory and claims a combined approach. Persistent epithelial defect is a pathology that, despite the fact that there are many treatments available for this condition [1–3], often cannot be resolved without

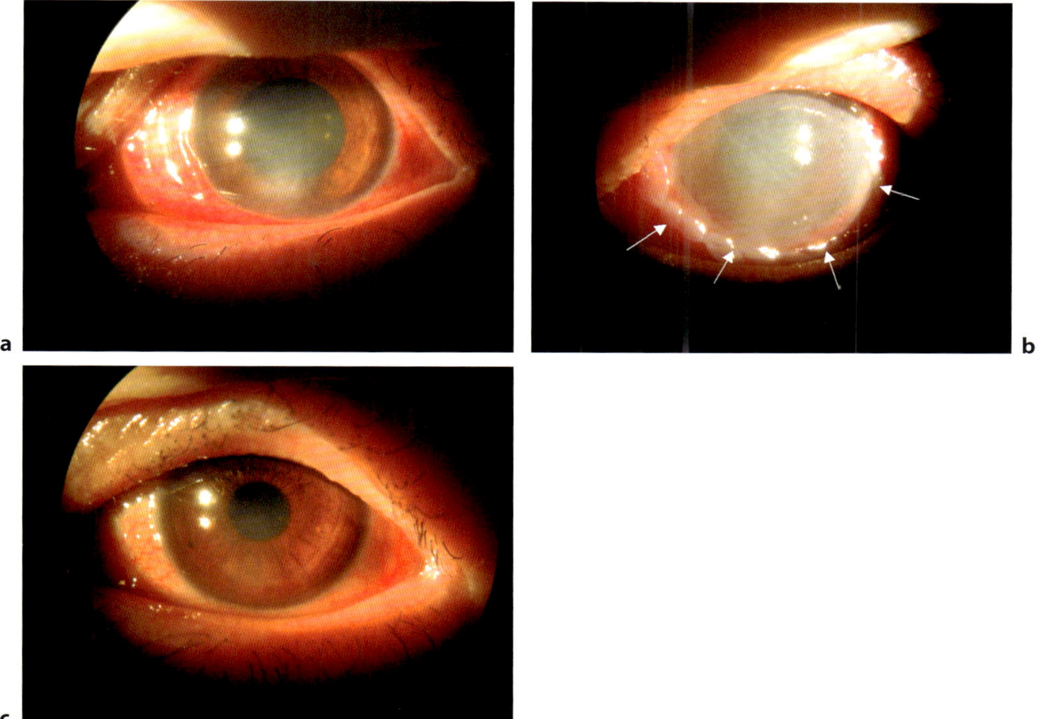

Fig. 2. **a** Persistent epithelial defect and stromal inflammation confined to one quadrant after corneal trauma. **b** The AM graft placed on the eye and secured with running 10-0 (Biosorb) sutures. The arrows define the edges of the graft. **c** Postoperative appearance after 3 months demonstrating a clear, epithelialized corneal surface.

amniotic membrane transplantation (AMT) [4–6] (fig. 2a–c). This syndrome usually arises following trauma of the corneal surface or as a result of anterior stromal dystrophy. Another indication for AMT to the anterior eye surface includes corneal ulceration with progressive thinning, descemetocoele and/or corneal perforation [7]. The most common cause for such conditions is corneal infection (fig. 3), but it can also be seen in auto-immune diseases, chronic inflammation or trauma. AMT in such diseases may allow final, reparative treatment by penetrating keratoplasty to be postponed until the eye becomes less inflamed. This is of special benefit for the patient since the outcome of penetrating keratoplasty will improve significantly when the surgery is performed in a non-inflamed eye. Prior to AMT, loose or necrotic tissue surrounding the ulcer should be removed and cultures taken (if there is concern about infection). In case of a very deep corneal ulcer, several layers of AM can be used to fill completely the crater formed by the ulcer. Those covered by the AM, both on the anterior eye surface and anterior chamber, will be harder to inspect, and the process of AM absorption takes approximately 4 weeks.

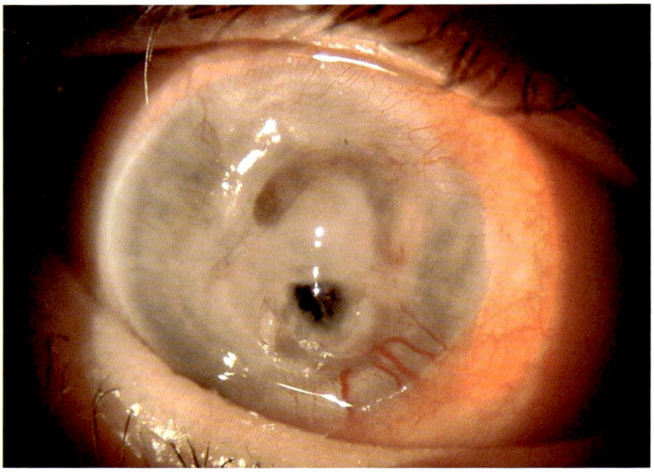

Fig. 3. Corneal ulceration with progressive thinning and descemtocoele due to the corneal infection. Penetrating keratoplasty in such an eye would have a high rejection rate; thus, AMT is indicated to fill the corneal defect and suppress ocular inflammation prior to penetrating keratoplasty.

Another treatment challenge is a recurrence-free pterygium surgery. For this degenerative ocular surface disorder with excessive fibrovascular tissue proliferation on the cornea, numerous surgical approaches have been attempted. Prior to the use of AM, the defect resulting after pterygium excision had been either exposed – 'bare sclera excision' – or covered by surrounding conjunctiva [8, 9]. When the 'bare sclera' technique is used, an adjunctive therapy such as beta radiation, thiotepa or mitomycin C is required to reduce the recurrence rate [10, 11]. It is well known that these adjunctive treatments are associated with complications such as superficial keratitis, poor epithelial healing, scleral ulceration and microbial infection [12]. Therefore conjunctival autografting has been widely adopted in the treatment of recurrent pterygia. But for those advanced pterygia, with wide conjunctival involvement, this procedure might be limited by the lack of remaining healthy tissue in the same or fellow eye. In such cases, AMT is recommended since a sufficient amount of substitute tissue can be provided regardless of the size of the bare sclera. Recent studies comparing the effect of AMT and limbal-conjunctival autograft show that conjunctival grafting is still a superior method in pterygium surgery; however, if the extent of bare sclera is too large to use this method, AMT is recommended [13].

There are several other ocular surface diseases where excision of diseased conjunctival tissue results in large portions of bare sclera, such as dysplasia, tumours, scars and symblepharon. After removal of a diseased conjunctiva, excessive formation of granulated tissue can take place, disfiguring the appearance and restricting the eyeball motility. To avoid this potential complication, autografts from the conjunctiva or the oral mucous membrane have been tried in eyes with huge conjunctival defects. Although a high success rate has been reported for these procedures, scarring of the donor tissue has been noted [14]. Therefore, AMT is used nowadays

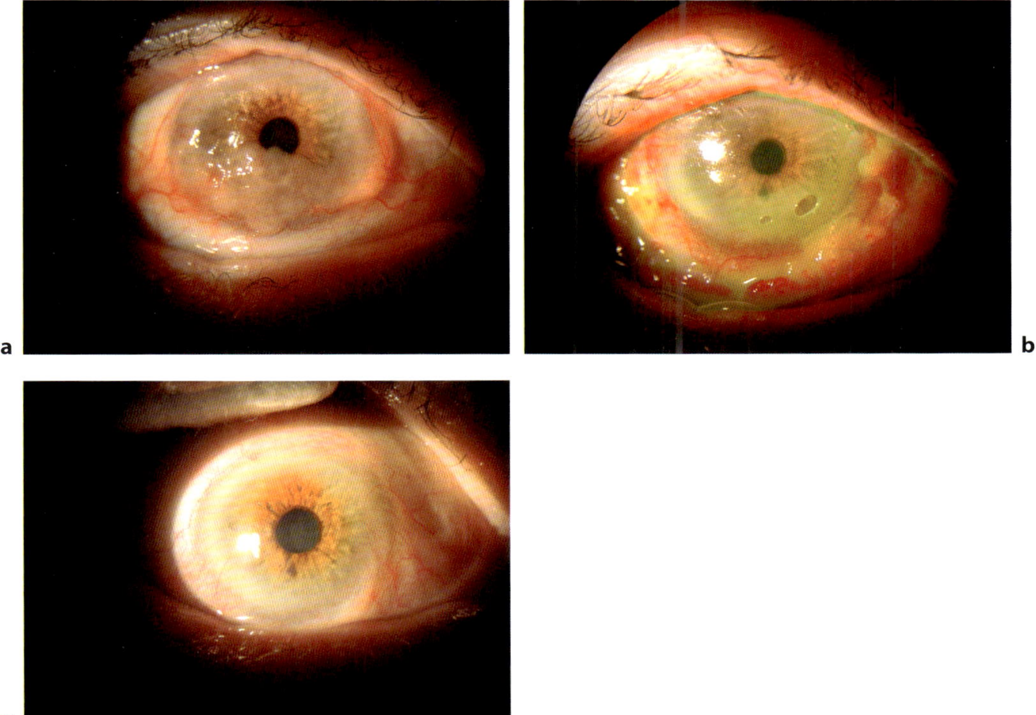

Fig. 4. **a** Pre-operative appearance of an eye with squamous cell carcinoma infiltrating a large portion of the corneal epithelial surface and surrounding conjunctiva. **b** Postoperative appearance 2 months after tumour removal and application of AM. AM is still covering the corneal surface. **c** Two years after excision of squamous cell carcinoma there is no sign of tumour regrowth or corneal scarring.

as a treatment option due to the properties of the AM: it facilitates migration and growth of epithelial cells and secretes anti-inflammatory and growth factors which prevent formation of vascularized granulation tissue and abundant scarring (fig. 4a–c). In the successful reconstruction, the epithelial cells cover the AM; conjunctival and corneal surfaces are stable, non-inflamed and free of neovascularization, although the exact mechanism achieving these results is still under investigation [15–17].

Chemical eye burns (especially with alkali) often lead to corneal blindness due to the loss of the normal ocular surface. Such injuries compromise the stem cell pool, causing partial or even total limbal stem cell deficiency. Stem cells, which are located in the basal layer of the limbal epithelium and held responsible for the maintenance of normal corneal epithelium, may be destroyed not only by the chemical burn itself, but also as a result of the consequent inflammatory destruction [18]. Several surgical strategies had been tried in patients with severe chemical burns that responded poorly to conservative treatment, either alone or combined: AMT, conjunctival limbal autograft or allograft transplantation and transplantation of limbal stem cells cultured ex vivo on the AM [19–23]. The beneficial effect of these procedures has been thought to result from a combination of immunosuppressive ability of the AM and substitution of destroyed limbal tissue. In case of total limbal stem cell deficiency, AM alone cannot correct an ocular surface disorder, and it should always be combined with a limbal autograft, while partial limbal stem cell deficiency can be solved with AMT alone. Successful surgical treatment results in corneal epithelialization, reduction of stromal opacity and neovascularization, and establishment of the conjunctival fornix (fig. 5a–e). For the optimal visual rehabilitation, however, several months after the initial procedure penetrating keratoplasty may be needed. The optimal patient selection and timing of all the mentioned surgical approaches are still under investigation.

Surgical Techniques

There are several surgical approaches for AMT, for example using the 'inlay' technique where the membrane serves as substrate for re-epithelialization or the 'overlay' technique where the membrane is used as biological contact lens placed over the entire cornea, limbus and perilimbal area [24]. Regarding the number of AM layers placed onto the eye, the surgical approach is also divided into a 'monolayer' and 'multilayer' technique [7]. When applied as a 'monolayer' the AM is applied as in the overlay technique; AM is spread over the entire ocular surface without folds or tears, and sutured by running 10-0 resorptive sutures (Biosorb). In case of multilayer AMT, the inner layer(s) of AM is used as in the inlay method. A typical example is in deep corneal defects (ulcers): several layers (1, 2 or even more) of AM are placed inside the ulcer to fill the defect and enhance the epithelialization over the AM. During the healing process, AM becomes a constitutive part of the corneal stroma and enhances healing of the corneal defect. Finally, the whole cornea and surrounding ocular surface are covered with the larger piece of the AM as in the overlay method.

AMT is performed under subconjunctival or peribulbar anaesthesia. If sutures are placed onto the cornea or limbus, 10-0 resorptive (or nylon) interrupted sutures may be used; if the membrane is secured to the conjunctiva or bare sclera, a 10-0 resorptive continuous suture is recommended. A soft contact lens is placed over the membrane at the end of the surgery. Patient check-up is recommended on the first postoperative day and then on a weekly basis. A well-adjusted AM will be flattened over the corneal surface and relatively transparent. AM will usually resolve after 4–6 weeks, during which period its therapeutic properties will enhance healing of the ocular surface disease.

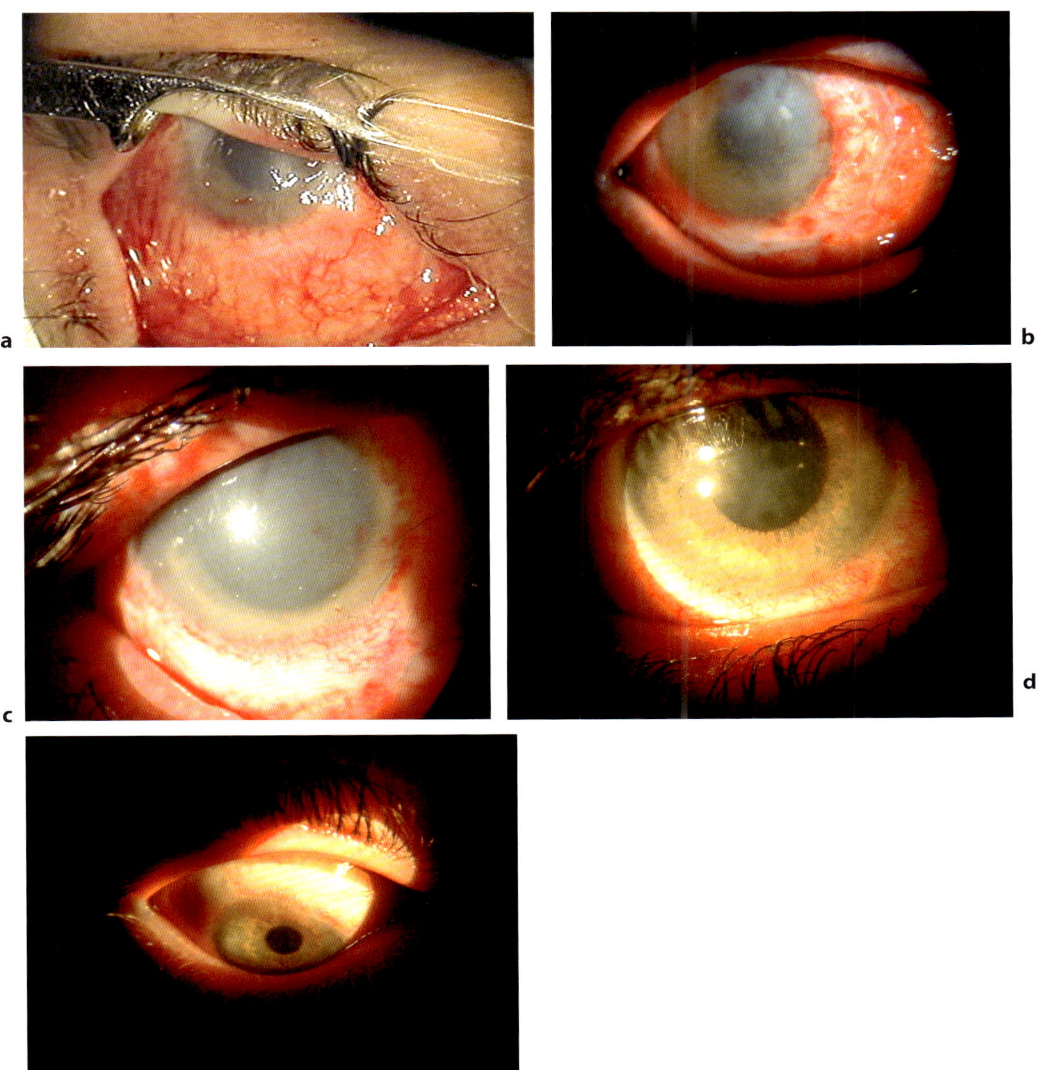

Fig. 5. a Signs of partial limbal stem cell deficiency in a patient that had sustained an alkali splash injury. The eye was initially treated by saline irrigation, topical steroid-antibiotic drops and prophylactic antibiotic coverage. An already formed symblepharon, persistent epithelial defect and corneal neovascularization were noted upon presentation (the lid speculum could not fit into the upper fornix). **b** The patient underwent multilayer AMT combined with symblepharolysis. The first AM layer was sized to fit the corneal defect and was secured with a running suture. The upper AM layer was placed to cover the entire cornea, adjacent to the bare sclera and superior fornix. The figure shows the appearance of the amniotic graft 3 days after surgery. The ocular surface shows reduced inflammation and movements of the bulb are free in all directions. **c** Postoperative appearance of the eye 3 weeks after multilayer AMT due to alkali burn. The upper AM layer is still in place, whilst remnants of the inner AM layer (seen as corneal opacities) appear to be integrated into the corneal stroma in places where the corneal basement membrane was damaged. **d**, **e** Fully epithelialized, clear and avascular cornea in the once heavily burned eye is the result of successful AMT. One year after surgery, the patient's uncorrected visual acuity is 20/20, and reformation of the upper fornix is fully visible at his down-gaze.

References

1 Ozkurt Y, Rodop O, Oral Y, Comez A, Kandemir B, Dogan OK: Therapeutic applications of lotrafilcon, a silicone hydrogel soft contact lens. Eye Contact Lens 2005;31:268–269.

2 Hondur A, Bilgihan K, Hasanreisoglu B: Phototherapeutic LASEK for a persistent epithelial defect and a recurrent epithelial erosion. J Refract Surg 2005;21:406–407.

3 Ramamurthi S, Ramaesh K: Anterior stromal puncture for recurrent corneal erosion after laser in situ keratomileusis. J Cataract Refract Surg 2005;31: 9–10.

4 Kim JC, Tseng SC: Transplantation of preserved human amniotic membrane for surface reconstruction in severely damaged rabbit corneas. Cornea 1995;14:473–484.

5 Gabric N, Mravicic I, Dekaris I, Karaman Z, Mitrovic S: Human amniotic membrane in the reconstruction of the ocular surface. Doc Ophthalmol 1999;98:273–283.

6 Tseng SC, Prabhasawat P, Lee SH: Amniotic membrane transplantation for conjunctival surface reconstruction. Am J Ophthalmol 1997;124:765–774.

7 Dekaris I, Gabric N, Mravicic I, Katusic J, Lazic R, Spoljaric N: Multilayer vs monolayer amniotic membrane transplantation for deep corneal ulcer treatment. Coll Antropol 2001;25(suppl):23–28.

8 Walkow T, Daniel J, Meyer CH, Rodrigues EB, Mennel S: Long-term results after bare sclera pterygium resection with excimer smoothing and local application of mitomycin C. Cornea 2005;24:378–381.

9 Miyai T, Hara R, Nejima R, Miyata K, Yonemura T, Amano S: Limbal allograft, amniotic membrane transplantation, and intraoperative mitomycin C for recurrent pterygium. Ophthalmology 2005;112:1263–1267.

10 Pajic B, Greiner RH: Long term results of non-surgical, exclusive strontium-/yttrium-90 beta-irradiation of pterygia. Radiother Oncol 2005;74:25–29.

11 Singh G, Wilson MR, Foster CS: Long term follow-up study of mitomycin eye drops as adjunctive treatment for pterygia and its comparison with conjunctival autograft transplantation. Cornea 1990;9:331–334.

12 Alsagoff Z, Tan DT, Chee SP: Necrotising scleritis after bare sclera excision of pterygium. Br J Ophthalmol 2000;84:1050–1052.

13 Dekaris I, Gabric N, Karaman Z, Mravicic I, Kastelan S, Spoljaric N: Pterygium treatment with limbal-conjunctival autograft transplantation. Coll Antropol 2001;25(suppl):7–12.

14 Vrabec MP, Weisienthal RW, Elsing SH: Subconjunctival fibrosis after conjunctival autograft. Cornea 1993;12:181–183.

15 Ueta M, Kweon MN, Sano Y, Sotozono C, Yamada J, Koizumi N, Kiyono H, Kinoshita S: Immunosuppressive properties of human amniotic membrane for mixed lymphocyte reaction. Clin Exp Immunol 2002;129:464–470.

16 Sotozono C, He J, Tei M, Honma Y, Kinoshita S: Effect of metalloproteinase inhibitor on corneal cytokine expression after alkali injury. Invest Ophthalmol Vis Sci 1999;40:2430–2434.

17 Shao C, Sima J, Zhang SX, Jin J, Reinach P, Wang Z, Ma JX: Suppression of corneal neovascularization by PEDF release from human amniotic membranes. Invest Ophthalmol Vis Sci 2004;45:1758–1762.

18 Lavker RM, Tseng SC, Sun TT: Corneal epithelial stem cells at the limbus: looking at some old problems from a new angle. Exp Eye Res 2004;78:433–446.

19 Gruterich M, Tseng SC: Surgical approaches for limbal stem cell deficiency. Klin Monatsbl Augenheilkd 2002;219:333–339.

20 Meallet MA, Espana EM, Grueterich M, Ti SE, Goto E, Tseng SC: Amniotic membrane transplantation with conjunctival limbal autograft for total limbal stem cell deficiency. Ophthalmology 2003;110:1585–1592.

21 Ozdemir O, Tekeli O, Ornek K, Arslanpence A, Yalcindag NF: Limbal autograft and allograft transplantations in patients with corneal burns. Eye 2004;18:241–248.

22 Shimazaki J, Aiba M, Goto E, Kato N, Shimmura S, Tsubota K: Transplantation of human limbal epithelium cultivated on amniotic membrane for the treatment of severe ocular surface disorders. Ophthalmology 2002;109:1285–1290.

23 Grueterich M, Tseng SC: Human limbal progenitor cells expanded on intact amniotic membrane ex vivo. Arch Ophthalmol 2002;120:783–790.

24 Kimberley CS, Foster S: Three pearls in amniotic membrane grafting; in Samir AM, Azar DT (eds): 101 Pearls in Refractive, Cataract and Corneal Surgery. Thorofare, Slack, 2001, pp 125–130.

Prof. Iva Dekaris, MD, PhD
Medical Director, Eye Clinic 'Svjetlost'
Heinzelova 39
HR–10000 Zagreb (Croatia)
E-Mail iva.dekaris@inet.hr

Bredehorn-Mayr T, Duncker GIW, Armitage WJ (eds): Eye Banking.
Dev Ophthalmol. Basel, Karger, 2009, vol 43, pp 105–108

Preparation and Use of Human Sclera Grafts in Ophthalmic Surgery

M. Töteberg-Harms[a,b] · T. Bredehorn-Mayr[b]

[a]Eye Clinic, University Hospital of Zurich, Zurich, Switzerland; [b]Eye Clinic, University Hospital of Halle, Halle (Saale), Germany

Abstract

Introduction: Human sclera grafts are widely used in ophthalmic surgery. Mainly they are used for coating orbital implants after enucleation. **Methods:** For the preparation of sclera grafts, all other tissues must be removed from the donor bulb including the retina, choroid, cornea, corpus vitreum and lens. The sclera graft can be stored dry or in ethanol until transplantation. **Results and Conclusion:** The processing of sclera grafts in an eye bank is easy to handle compared to the complexity of cornea transplants. The common way is dry storing for at least 1 year. Thus, the demand for sclera grafts can be covered without a lot of trouble.

Human sclera grafts are widely used in ophthalmic surgery. They are mainly used for coating orbital implants [1, 2] after enucleation, covering scleral damage [3, 4] as in rheumatoid arthritis or in reconstruction after complicated filtering bleb surgery [5] in glaucoma and in combination with buckling surgery [6]. Other examples include the covering of filtration systems such as an Ahmed valve [7] or in complex lid reconstructions [8, 9]. Coating orbital implants with human sclera allografts reduces the risk of rejection by the recipient.

Because the number of cornea donors far outweighs the demand for sclera grafts, there is no problem in getting as many sclera grafts as needed for a well-working eye bank. There may be a problem if an eye bank is predominantly removing only the corneoscleral discs instead of the whole bulbs from the donors. The removal of the bulb is described elsewhere in the chapter on corneal donation [this vol., pp. 22–30].

Methods

For the preparation of sclera grafts, first the whole conjunctiva and all muscles must be removed from the human donor bulb (fig. 1). Typically this has been done before the corneoscleral disc has

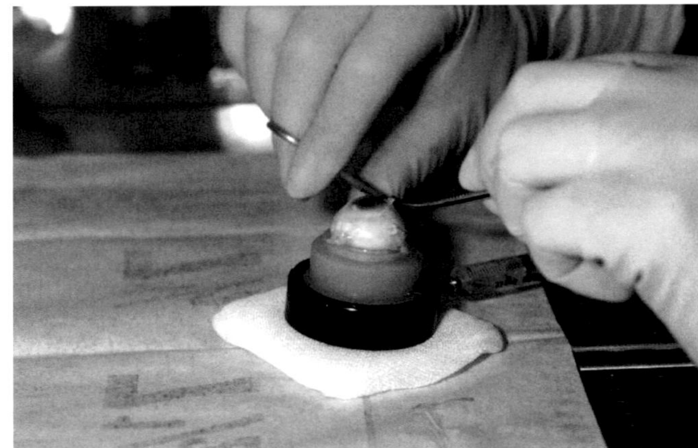

Fig. 1. Preparation of the bulb – removal of conjunctiva, Tenon's capsule and muscles.

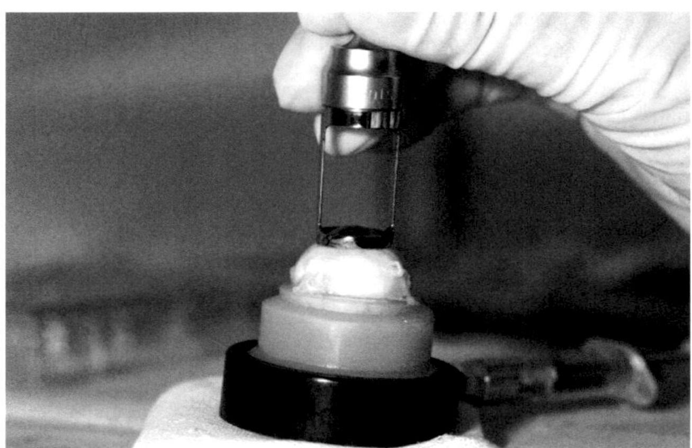

Fig. 2. Removing the corneoscleral disc by a trepine.

been removed by a trepine (fig. 2). Afterwards the whole content of the bulb – lens, corpus vitreum, retina and choroid – must be removed. This could easily be done by everting the bulb and cleaning the remains by scratching with a hockey knife on the inner side, which is now outside (fig. 3). At the end, the sclera graft can be stored until needed for transplantation.

Different methods for storage of sclera grafts in the eye bank have been established. The first way is storing the sclera graft in 90% ethanol (fig. 4) for prolonged periods of time at between 4 and 8°C (i.e. 39.2–46.4°F) without any further pretreatment. However, the most common method is dry storage. The sclera must first be deposited in 70% ethanol for 5 h followed by another 24 h in 96% ethanol. Afterwards, the graft has to be cleaned by sterile isotonic NaCl solution. To complete the process, the sclera is then dried by using, for example, the rest warmth of a hot air sterilizer. The sclera graft can then be stored for at least 1 year in a sterile tube in a refrigeration unit (fig. 5).

Before transplantation, the sclera grafts must again be processed. Using a solution of gentamycin is common (mix 40 mg of gentamycin with 10 ml 0.9% NaCl solution) for both methods of storage. If the graft is stored dry, it must be soaked in the gentamycin solution for at least 1 or 2 h. However, before doing this, we suggest getting a microbial smear of the dry transplant. If the graft is stored in

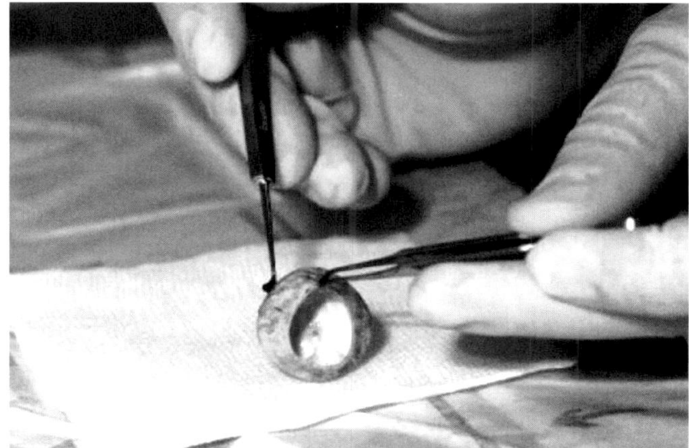

Fig. 3. Cleaning the inner side of the sclera by scratching with a hockey knife.

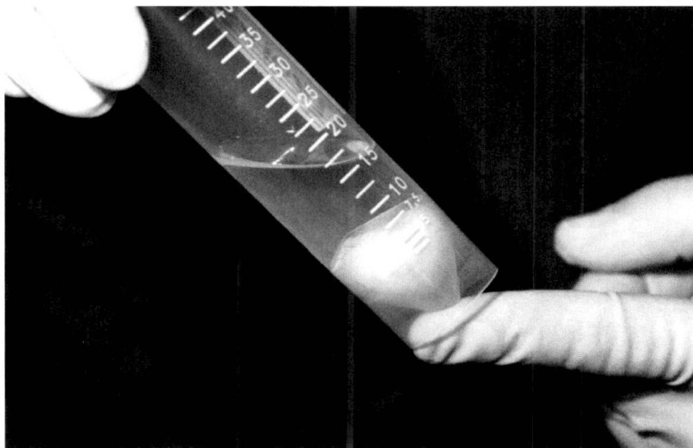

Fig. 4. Storage of a sclera graft in ethanol.

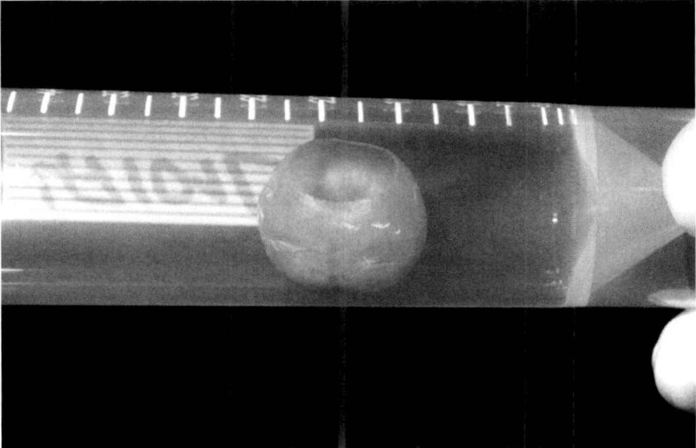

Fig. 5. Dry storage of a sclera graft in a Falcon™ tube.

ethanol, it must be soaked in the gentamycin solution for at least 2 h. The solution should be replaced once after the first hour.

Results and Conclusion

The preparation and storage of human sclera grafts are very easy. Yet, there is only less extra work if corneas are prepared for transplantation in an eye bank. The demand is also easily covered. We suggest to freeze the bulbs after trepanation of the corneoscleral grafts and to prepare a number of sclera grafts at one time (may be 4 times a year), storing them until needed for transplantation.

References

1 Georgiadis NS, Terzidou CD, Dimitriadis AS: Corraline hydroxyapatite sphere in orbit restoration. Eur J Ophthalmol 1999;9:302–308.

2 Kawai S, Suzuki T, Kawai K: Mobility of hydroxyapatite orbital implant covered with autologous sclera. Jpn J Ophthalmol 2000;44:68–74.

3 Lin CP, et al: Repair of giant sclera ulcer with preserved sclera and tissue adhesive. Ophthalmic Surg Lasers 1996;27:995–999.

4 Rodriguez-Ares MT, et al: Repair of scleral perforation with preserved scleral and amniotic membrane in Marfan's syndrome. Ophthalmic Surg Lasers 1999;30:485–487.

5 Aslanides IM, Spaeth GL, et al: Autologous patch graft in tube shunt surgery. J Glaucoma 1999;8:306–309.

6 Murdoch GR, Sampath R, et al: Autogenous labial mucous membrane and banked scleral patch grafting for exposed retinal explants. Eye 1997;11:43–46.

7 Rai P, Lauande-Pimentel R, Barton K: Amniotic membrane as an adjunct to donor sclera in the repair of exposed glaucoma drainage devices. Am J Ophthalmol 2005;140:148–152.

8 Olliver JM, Rose GE, et al: Correction of lower eyelid retraction in thyroid eye desease: a randomised controlled trial of retractor tenotomy with adjuvant antimetabolite versus scleral graft. Br J Ophthalmol 1998;82:174–180.

9 Kadoi C, Hayasaka S, et al: The Cutler-Beard bridge technique with use of donor sclera for upper eyelid reconstruction. Ophthalmologica 2000;214:140–142.

M. Töteberg-Harms
Eye Clinic
University Hospital of Zurich
CH–8032 Zurich (Switzerland)
Tel. +41 44 255 5940, Fax +41 44 255 44 38, E-Mail marc.toeteberg@usz.ch

Bredehorn-Mayr T, Duncker GIW, Armitage WJ (eds): Eye Banking.
Dev Ophthalmol. Basel, Karger, 2009, vol 43, pp 109–119

Culturing of Retinal Pigment Epithelium Cells

Monika Valtink[a] · Katrin Engelmann[b,c]

[a]Institute of Anatomy, Medical Faculty 'Carl Gustav Caris', TU Dresden, [b]CRTD/DFG-Center for Regenerative Therapies Dresden – Cluster of Excellence, Dresden, and [c]Department of Ophthalmology, Städtisches Klinikum Chemnitz gGmbH, Chemnitz, Germany

Abstract

The retinal pigment epithelium (RPE) is a monolayer of cells adjacent to the photoreceptors of the retina. It plays a crucial role in maintaining photoreceptor health and survival. Degeneration or dysfunction of the RPE can lead to photoreceptor degeneration and as a consequence to visual impairment. The most common diseased state of the RPE becomes manifest in age-related macular degeneration, an increasing cause of blindness in the elderly. RPE cells are therefore of great interest to researchers working in the field of tissue engineering and cell transplantation. In fact, studies in animal models have proven that the transplantation of RPE cells can delay the course of photoreceptor degenerative diseases. Although first attempts to transplant RPE cells into the subretinal space in human individuals suffering from age-related macular degeneration were less successful, RPE cell transplantation is still favored as a future therapeutic option, and much work is done to develop and design cell transplants. Cell banking is a prerequisite to have well-differentiated and characterized cells at hand when needed for research purposes, but also for therapeutic approaches. In this chapter the authors will describe methods to isolate, culture and preserve adult human RPE cells for the purpose of RPE cell banking.

The Retinal Pigment Epithelium

The retinal pigment epithelium (RPE) forms a monolayer of heavily pigmented, polygonal cells. It resides between the neurosensory retina and the choroid, and represents part of the blood-retina barrier. RPE cells are polarized and function as a transport epithelium. The polarized structure results from the differential expression of proteins on the apical side facing the retina and the basolateral side facing the choroid. This polarized structure allows a directional transport of fluids, nutrients and metabolic waste products between the retina and choroid through junctional complexes between the RPE cells. Furthermore the RPE accounts for dehydration of the subretinal space. Its main function is to supply the adjacent photoreceptor cells with nutrients and to remove photoreceptor outer segments, which are shed daily in a circadian rhythm. These outer segments are phagocytosed, metabolized and removed via the adjacent choroidal blood vessels. By this the RPE also participates in the retinoid cycle to recover visual pigments, namely rhodopsin [1].

Retinal Pigment Epithelium in Cell Culture

The in vitro cultivation of primary, i.e. nontransfected or nontransformed, cells especially of human origin is a complex and demanding task. This holds all the more true for terminally differentiated and postmitotic cells like those of the RPE. Detailed protocols for isolation and cultivation are required in order to meet the specific needs of such cells, and they may vary considerably with respect to the cell type of interest. Culturing ocular cells is furthermore challenging, because the initial number of cells that can be isolated is limited due to the small size of the eye, and quite a few ocular cell types that are interesting for e.g. tissue engineering purposes appear in monolayers. As a rule, these cells can only be isolated from postmortem tissue, which limits their viability and further decreases the number of cultivable cells. Except for some few ocular progenitor cells that have been characterized in recent years [2, 3], most types of ocular cells are generally terminally differentiated and postmitotic in vivo, which means that proliferation in vitro resembles an atypical state. The cells have to re-enter the cell cycle, and this may lead not only to proliferation, but also to a loss of differentiated characteristics, since differentiation of these cells is basically linked to cell cycle arrest. The use of elaborated and refined cell culture protocols can help to minimize such de- or transdifferentiation.

First attempts to culture RPE cells go back to the 60s, and in 1972 Albert et al. [4] were the first to describe in detail the growth behavior of choroidal explants in culture. Since then various techniques to isolate and cultivate RPE cells in consideration of proliferation and cell morphology were investigated, e.g. Pfeffer [5] isolated the cells using dispase after fenestration of the sclera. Flood et al. [6] and Baumgartner et al. [7] removed the anterior segment and vitreous, and filled the remaining eyecup with trypsin or incubated the choroid in trypsin after mechanical removal. Such procedures yielded single cells as well as cell clusters. Various basal media were used for cultivation, e.g. RPMI 1640 [4, 7], minimal essential medium (MEM) [8] or medium 199 [9], all usually supplemented with 10–20% serum. Only rarely were other supplements like insulin or bicarbonate [10] added. In 1991, Pfeffer [5] described the development of a specific culture medium for primate and human RPE cells, which can be used in two slightly different compositions either for promoting proliferation or for inducing differentiation of the cultured cells. Despite all these attempts, until now, there has been no uniform or standardized method to isolate and culture RPE cells.

It could be observed that RPE cells show a strong tendency to dedifferentiate during in vitro cultivation, which becomes manifest in marked morphological changes [11]. RPE cells in higher passages usually develop a fibroblastoid phenotype, but changes towards a myoid phenotype were also described [12]. Such metaplastic alterations of the RPE were also observed in some disease patterns, e.g. proliferative vitreoretinopathy.

Most experiments dealing with RPE cells in vitro were performed to study cellular behavior and specific RPE functions, or to elucidate signal transduction pathways or effects of growth and survival factors [1]. Another experimental field for use of primary RPE cells and sometimes also cell lines is studying the toxicity of substances or conditions which are estimated to have a deteriorating effect on the retina, e.g. staining substances to facilitate macular surgery or light-induced toxicity [13–17]. In addition, with regard to age-related macular degeneration as a major cause for vision impairment in the western world, transplantation of RPE cells was studied extensively in animal models [18] and furthermore also as a therapeutic approach for Parkinson's disease [19]. The transplantation of RPE cells as a therapy can only be successful if the graft cells retain their differentiated morphology and functionality. To achieve this, specifically designed cell culture protocols are needed, which meet the requirements of RPE cells and resemble as much as possible their in vivo microenvironment.

However, such a detailed elaboration of culture protocols for RPE cells has so far only been described by Pfeffer [5], who was e.g. using retinal extract as one of the key supplements to supply the cells with specific nutrients. Most experiments were performed under standard culture conditions including supplementation of the medium with serum. Serum is known to increase cell proliferation and survival of the cells, but RPE cells undergo rapid morphological changes under proliferation-stimulating conditions (dedifferentiation or deadaptation). Furthermore, working with serum bears the risk of masking effects of the substances to be investigated in cell culture. Results obtained from serum-supplemented cultures may therefore not correspond with signals from differentiated RPE cells. If cells are cultured for subsequent transplantation purposes, serum should be avoided to minimize the risk of transferring animal pathogens.

Optimizing Retinal Pigment Epithelium Cell Cultivation

Isolation Techniques

The cultivation methods described in the literature as well as our own studies confirmed that differentiation of the cells can be maintained over several passages by optimizing the isolation and cultivation procedures. These studies report the expression of highly differentiated proteins like bestrophin or polarized expression of Na-K-ATPase, as well as the expression of certain ion channel proteins after passaging and cryopreservation when cells were cultured under improved conditions [20, 21]. The composition of the culture medium is of particular importance in order to successfully establish primary cell cultures. The choice of medium components and the kind of supplements as well as their concentration have a demonstrable influence upon viability, morphology and proliferative capacity of the in vitro cultured cells. Besides the protein and lipid fraction of the medium and the hormone content, low-molecular-weight substances like salts, sugars or vitamins also play a critical role.

Experiments to improve the isolation of RPE cells from human cadaveric eyes with longer postmortem times revealed that high numbers of cells could be obtained when using trypsin. However, the impaired viability of cells from postmortem eyes was derogated further by the nonselective proteolytic activity of this enzyme so that only about 1% of the cells were vital enough to survive the isolation procedure and eventually start a growing cell culture [22]. Although the incubation of the RPE-choroid complex in dispase, another but milder nonselective proteolytic enzyme, has been reported as an efficient method to isolate RPE cells [23, 24], according to our experience dispase treatment yields a high number of co-isolated, contaminating choroidal melanocytes that usually overgrow the few isolated RPE cells. A gentle but effective enzymatic treatment of the choroidal sheets with a mixture of collagenase IA and collagenase IV instead of trypsin or dispase yields almost pure RPE cell cultures (fig. 1). The cells cultured after isolation with the collagenase mixture grew remarkably faster than cells cultured after isolation with trypsin or dispase, as concluded from the duration from isolation until confluence of the culture [22]. Besides testing various enzymes, the two aforementioned techniques to access the RPE layer were tried out as well: both methods require to remove the anterior segment, vitreous and neurosensory retina, but while according to Flood et al. [6] the eyecup is filled with enzyme solution, the method according to Baumgartner et al. [7] requires preparing the choroid-RPE complex off the sclera with forceps and scissors and incubation of the sheets in enzyme solution. It was observed that the second method seems advantageous, since the choroidal sheets show a tendency to detach from the sclera and to collapse when left in the eyecup, most likely because of decomposing processes due to longer postmortem times so that filling the eyecup with enzyme solution becomes difficult.

Substrates and Matrices

RPE cells are adherent cells that reside on a basal lamina. In vivo and in vitro RPE cells produce an extracellular matrix (ECM), which is composed of mainly laminin, fibronectin, collagens I and IV and vitronectin, and the cells bind to these molecules with integrins [25]. A critical point in culturing RPE cells is how quickly the cells can adhere to the culture dish. Studies by Tezel and Del Priore [26] have shown that, depending on the attachment rate, RPE cells tend to undergo apoptosis if cell attachment is hampered. The soluble factors supplied with the medium, e.g. serum-derived vitronectin, are insufficiently mediating attachment so that additional coating of the culture dishes is necessary. Depending on the kind of substratum supplied to the cells, adherence is mediated more or less effectively [26, 27]. Furthermore, the kind

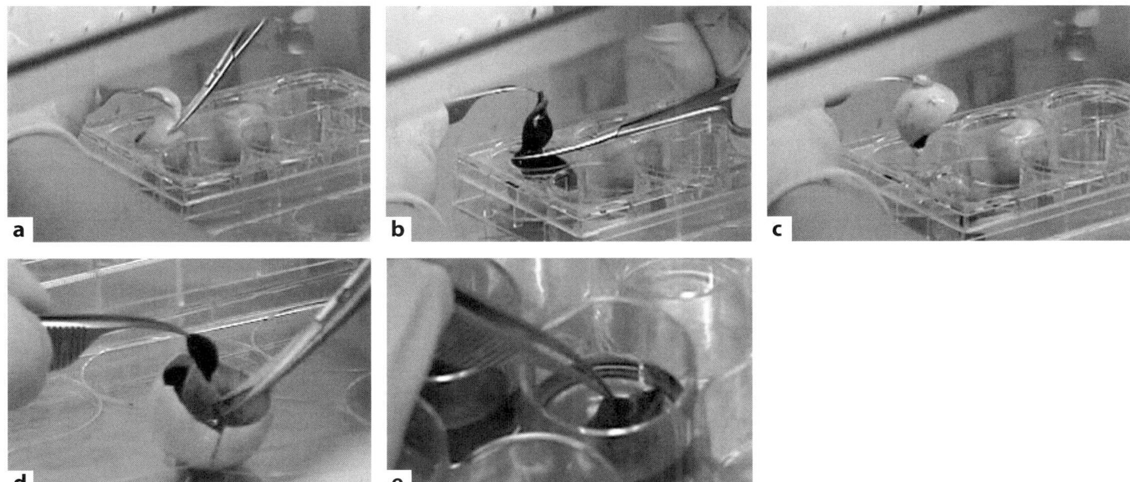

Fig. 1. Preparation of choroidal sheets for RPE cell isolation. **a** After removal of the cornea with a 15-mm trephine, the scleral opening is enlarged by circumferential cutting. **b** Iris and lens are removed. **c** The vitreous is poured out. **d** After removal of the neural retina, the choroidal sheet is prepared with scissors and fine forceps. Cutting the eye bulb into two halves may facilitate choroid preparation. **e** The choroidal sheets are transferred to a collagenase solution, unfolded with fine forceps and then incubated to release RPE cells.

of substratum has also an extensive regulatory influence on adhesion, proliferation, differentiation and also chemotactic behavior of the cells, since specific integrin binding to the ECM or provided protein substrates initiates defined signal transduction cascades [23, 24, 28–30].

In cell culture, ECM or its single components can be used to coat culture dishes in order to facilitate attachment and ensure survival of the plated cells. ECM can easily be produced by lysing the cells of postconfluent cultures (normally about 2 weeks confluent) carefully with 0.25% NH_4OH. The remaining ECM can be kept under PBS at 4°C for up to 2 weeks. ECM produced by corneal endothelial cells, e.g. porcine or bovine, shows the best attachment results, but ECM produced by fibroblast cell lines has also been proven to be efficient. However, the coating of dishes with naturally grown ECM is time-consuming and bears a higher risk of contamination. If RPE cells are cultured for subsequent transplantation procedures, it has to be considered that the ECM is produced by cells from another donor or even another species. A complete lysis of these cells cannot be assured, as some producer cells may survive the lysing step and may then contaminate the RPE culture. To avoid this risk, culture dishes can also be coated with single purified matrix proteins such as collagen, laminin or fibronectin. However, if RPE cell cultivation is to be performed as a routine procedure or at a large scale, the costs of coating dishes have to be considered, and instead of expensive ECM proteins substrates such as Matrigel or gelatin provide a cost-efficient alternative.

Culture Medium

In addition to a suitable isolation technique, the choice of an appropriate culture medium is of relevance in order to successfully establish a cell culture. Already the basal medium exerts a marked influence on the cells, as could be shown by Karl et al. [31], who demonstrated the tremendous effects basal media and supplements can exert on the phagocytic activity as a major function of RPE cells. In comparative experiments, several basal media or their 1/1 mixtures were tested regarding their ability to promote proliferation of human RPE cells in vitro, namely Ham's F12, medium 199(E), MEM-α and MEM. Best results were achieved with F99, a 1/1 mixture of Ham's F12 and medium 199, which was already shown to be suitable for cultivating other ocular cells [32]. By studying the effects of various supplements to F99, a growth medium specifically composed to promote growth of human RPE cells was developed, called $F99_{RPE}$ [22].

One of the main components of this growth medium is choroid-conditioned medium, which is prepared by incubating the choroidal remnants (after enzymatic isolation of RPE cells) in medium F99 + 1% fetal calf serum for 4 days [20]. It is known that conditioned media contain growth factors that are secreted by the cells during the conditioning process. However, conditioned media are undefined supplements, because their composition remains unknown. Their beneficial effect on proliferation and often also on differentiation of in vitro cultured cells is proven. The use of such an optimized cultivation protocol gives rise to an improved growth of primary human RPE cells and also the maintenance of some differentiated features of the cultured cells during subcultivation and cryopreservation [20].

Substitution of Serum in the Culture Medium

Nowadays, the reduction of serum or its replacement by defined single substances in the culture medium seems inevitable for several reasons, since bovine serum is regarded as a potential source of pathogens like bovine spongiform encephalopathy. This applies especially when cells are cultured for transplantation purposes or tissue engineering, a research field that is growing extensively. Even more important concerning cultivation is the fact that serum is associated with several disadvantages: lots vary in quality, its composition is unknown, future limitation of sources, economic and ethical reasons. Testing of basal media suitable for use without serum supplementation can easily be performed using growth assays, which are proven to be a valuable tool in cell culture optimization and which can be used to even detect the smallest differences between media and supplements [32, 33]. Growth and survival factors that can promote proliferation and/or differentiation of the cells are most suitable to substitute for serum. For RPE cells, basic fibroblast growth factor can play such a dual role in that it acts as a potent mitogen, but also supports the maintenance of a differentiated state of the cells in vitro [34]. Likewise, it could

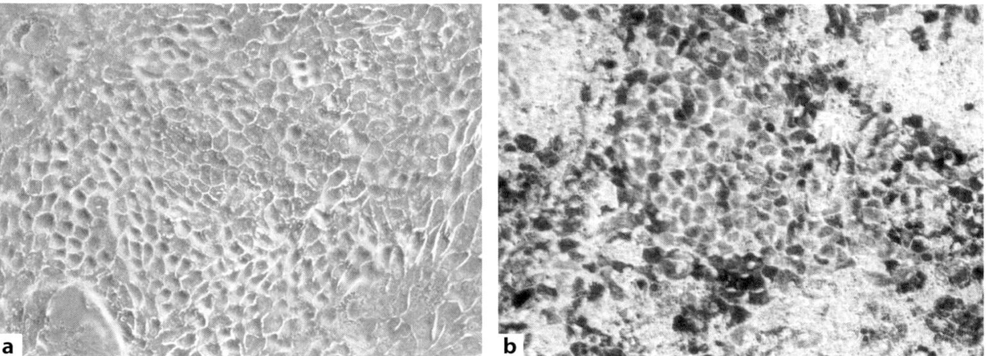

Fig. 2. Human adult RPE cells in culture, showing a polygonal epithelioid morphology: unpigmented (**a**) and pigmented (**b**).

be shown that other factors such as epidermal growth factor, vascular growth factor and platelet-derived growth factor exert an effect on cultured RPE cells [8, 12, 34–40].

Other substances that influence the proliferation, morphology or functional efficiency of RPE cells in vitro are bicarbonate [10], pyruvate [22], retinoic acid as well as hormones like insulin [10, 22], hydrocortisone [5] and transferrin. As an example, we like to restate the defined medium developed by Pfeffer [5], which can be used in two slightly different formulations to either promote proliferation or differentiation of RPE cells. These two formulations differ mainly in their concentration of low-molecular-weight molecules such as sodium pyruvate or calcium, but also in the supplementation of retinal extract. His studies show that continuous adaptation of cell culture protocols to the specific needs of the cells plays a vital role in the success of in vitro cell cultivation of RPE cells. Other groups have also described the successful use of serum-reduced or serum-free culture conditions to establish and serially passage RPE cells [21, 41]. These media were successfully developed in order to minimize serum-related morphological and functional alterations of RPE cells in vitro.

In several studies using human corneal endothelial cells and whole corneas, we found that a commercially available serum-free medium (human endothelial serum-free medium) exerted a beneficial effect on the growth and morphology of corneal endothelial cells [42, 43]. We tested this medium also on human RPE cells in vitro, because we had observed in previous experiments that corneal endothelial cells and RPE cells seem to have similar nutrient requirements [31, 44]. Like in serum supplementation culture, the serum-free cultured RPE cells initially lost their pigmentation but regained highly differentiated features such as a hexagonal morphology (fig. 2) with phase-bright cell borders and proper expression of tight junction proteins, de novo melanogenesis as proven by Hmb-45 staining and de novo RPE65 expression.

Although the cells showed a markedly reduced growth capacity, cultures could be maintained for several months [45].

Cryopreservation

Like other human and animal cells, RPE cells can easily be stored cryopreserved according to standard cell culture protocols. The best survival rates will be achieved when cells are cryopreserved in fetal calf serum supplemented with 10% dimethylsulfoxide as a cryoprotectant. However, if cells are cultured serum-free, the cryomedium should also be serum-free. For this, ready-to-use serum-free cryomedia are commercially available from different companies. The most widely used method to freeze cells is to use a protocol with a cooling rate of –1°C/min down to –80°C and subsequent transfer into liquid nitrogen. This protocol can easily be applied to RPE cells. It should be noted that cells which are cryopreserved under serum-free conditions are more sensitive towards temperature gradients than cells kept in fetal calf serum. When the freezing protocol mentioned above is applied to RPE cells, the cell sample should not be kept at –80°C for a longer time but should be transferred into liquid nitrogen as soon as possible; otherwise, the survival rate of the cells may decline markedly.

Retinal Pigment Epithelium Cell Banking and the Use of Cell Lines

The idea of RPE cell banking arose at a time when much hope was pinned on the transplantation of RPE cells in cases of age-related macular degeneration [18, 46–48]. Banking and preservation of primary RPE cells for tissue engineering is laborious and requires long-term preservation of the cells according to adapted culture conditions. But cell banking is more than developing optimum culture and storage conditions: it involves specific logistic and documentational efforts. This highly demanding task can only be met under professional organizational structures. Even though first attempts to transplant RPE cells in patients did not yield the expected results, it remains important to intensify research efforts in this direction. Moreover, the task of such cell banks can be the development, handling and characterization of cell lines for research approaches, because cell lines may replace fresh or primary RPE cell cultures in scientific experiments. Such cell lines should be carefully characterized regarding their specific function and differentiation capability. A widely used cell line is ARPE-19 [49], but SV40-transfected RPE cell lines like the one established in our laboratory are also intensively studied [31, 50].

As stated before, it is important to work with RPE cells that have a high differentiation degree in order to develop a cell transplantation therapy, e.g. for patients with age-related macular degeneration, because results obtained from experiments performed with deadapted/dedifferentiated and fibroblastoid or even myofibroblastoid

RPE cells may not reflect actual healthy RPE cell behavior. Not every laboratory can render services to elaborate and establish culture protocols that are adjusted to all cell types used. It seems more sensible to turn this task over to cell banks that will do such preliminary work for research groups. With respect to novel amendments and changes in legislation and guidelines on the handling of human cells and tissues, this aspect may gain in importance.

References

1 Marmor MF, Wolfensberger TJ (eds): The Retinal Pigment Epithelium: Function and Disease. New York, Oxford University Press, 1998.

2 Vascotto SG, Griffith M: Localization of candidate stem and progenitor cell markers within the human cornea, limbus, and bulbar conjunctiva in vivo and in cell culture. Anat Rec A 2006;288A:921–931.

3 Coles BL, Angenieux B, Inoue T, Del Rio-Tsonis K, Spence JR, McInnes RR, Arsenijevic Y, van der Kooy D: Facile isolation and the characterization of human retinal stem cells. Proc Natl Acad Sci USA 2004;101:15772–15777.

4 Albert DM, Tso MO, Rabson AS: In vitro growth of pure cultures of retinal pigment epithelium. Arch Ophthalmol 1972;88:63–69.

5 Pfeffer B: Improved methodology for cell culture of human and monkey retinal pigment epithelium. Prog Retinal Res 1991;10:251–291.

6 Flood MT, Gouras P, Kjeldbye H: Growth characteristics and ultrastructure of human retinal pigment epithelium in vitro. Invest Ophthalmol Vis Sci 1980; 19:1309–1320.

7 Baumgartner I, Huber-Spitzy V, Grabner G, Mayr WR: HLA typing from human donor eyes. Graefes Arch Clin Exp Ophthalmol 1989;227:541–543.

8 Adamis AP, Shima DT, Yeo KT, Yeo TK, Brown LF, Berse B, D'Amore PA, Folkman J: Synthesis and secretion of vascular permeability factor/vascular endothelial growth factor by human retinal pigment epithelial cells. Biochem Biophys Res Commun 1993;193:631–638.

9 Giordano GG, Thomson RC, Ishaug SL, Mikos AG, Cumber S, Garcia CA, Lahiri-Munir D: Retinal pigment epithelium cells cultured on synthetic biodegradable polymers. J Biomed Mater Res 1997;34: 87–93.

10 Kurtz MJ, Edwards RB: Influence of bicarbonate and insulin on pigment synthesis by cultured adult human retinal pigment epithelial cells. Exp Eye Res 1991;53:681–684.

11 MacDonald C: Primary culture and the establishment of cell lines; in Davis JM (ed): Basic Cell Culture: A Practical Approach. Oxford, IRL Press, 1994, pp 149–180.

12 Grisanti S, Esser P, Schraermeyer U: Retinal pigment epithelial cells: autocrine and paracrine stimulation of extracellular matrix contraction. Graefes Arch Clin Exp Ophthalmol 1997;235:587–598.

13 Algvere PV, Marshall J, Seregard S Age-related maculopathy and the impact of blue light hazard. Acta Ophthalmol Scand 2006;84:4–15

14 Cheng SN, Yang TC, Ho JD, Hwang JF, Cheng CK: Ocular toxicity of intravitreal indocyanine green. J Ocul Pharmacol Ther 2005;21:85–93.

15 Gandorfer A, Haritoglou C, Gandorfer A, Kampik A: Retinal damage from indocyanine green in experimental macular surgery. Invest Ophthalmol Vis Sci 2003;44:316–323.

16 Haritoglou C, Priglinger S, Gandorfer A, Welge-Lussen U, Kampik A: Histology of the vitreoretinal interface after indocyanine green staining of the ILM, with illumination using a halogen and xenon light source. Invest Ophthalmol Vis Sci 2005;46: 1468–1472.

17 Whitehead AJ, Mares JA, Danis RP: Macular pigment – a review of current knowledge. Arch Ophthalmol 2006;124:1038–1045.

18 Valtink M, Weichel J, Richard G, Engelmann K: Transplantation of retinal pigment epithelium cells; in Alberti W, Richard G, Sagerman R (eds): Age-Related Macular Degeneration: Current Treatment Concepts. Berlin, Springer, 2001, pp 65–76.

19 Doudet DJ, Cornfeldt ML, Honey CR, Schweikert AW, Allen RC: PET imaging of implanted human retinal pigment epithelial cells in the MPTP-induced primate model of Parkinson's disease. Exp Neurol 2004;189:361–368.

20 Valtink M, Engelmann K, Strauss O, Kruger R, Loliger C, Ventura AS, Richard G: Physiological features of primary cultures and subcultures of human retinal pigment epithelial cells before and after cryopreservation for cell transplantation. Graefes Arch Clin Exp Ophthalmol 1999;237:1001–1006.

21 Hu J, Bok D: A cell culture medium that supports the differentiation of human retinal pigment epithelium into functionally polarized monolayers. Mol Vis 2000;7:14–19.
22 Sobottka Ventura AC, Bohnke M, Loliger C, Kuhnl P, Winter R, Engelmann K: HLA typing of donor corneas with extended post mortem time (in German). Ophthalmologe 1996;93:262–267.
23 Opas M, Dziak E: Effects of substrata and method of tissue dissociation on adhesion, cytoskeleton, and growth of chick retinal pigmented epithelium in vitro. In Vitro Cell Dev Biol 1988;24:885–892.
24 Tezel TH, Del Priore LV, Kaplan HJ: Harvest and storage of adult human retinal pigment epithelial sheets. Curr Eye Res 1997;16:802–809.
25 Ho TC, Del Priore LV: Reattachment of cultured human retinal pigment epithelium to extracellular matrix and human Bruch's membrane. Invest Ophthalmol Vis Sci 1997;38:1110–1118.
26 Tezel TH, Del Priore LV: Reattachment to a substrate prevents apoptosis of human retinal pigment epithelium. Graefes Arch Clin Exp Ophthalmol 1997;235:41–47.
27 Newsome DA, Pfeffer BA, Hewitt AT, Robey PG, Hassell JR: Detection of extracellular matrix molecules synthesized in vitro by monkey and human retinal pigment epithelium: influence of donor age and multiple passages. Exp Eye Res 1988;46:305–321.
28 Campochiaro PA, Jerdon JA, Glaser BM: The extracellular matrix of human retinal pigment epithelial cells in vivo and its synthesis in vitro. Invest Ophthalmol Vis Sci 1986;27:1615–1621.
29 Docherty RJ, Forrester JV, Lackie JM: Type I collagen permits invasive behaviour by retinal pigmented epithelial cells in vitro. J Cell Sci 1987;87:399–409.
30 Strauss O, Wienrich M: Extracellular matrix proteins as substrate modulate the pattern of calcium channel expression in cultured rat retinal pigment epithelial cells. Pflugers Arch 1994;429:137–139.
31 Karl MO, Valtink M, Bednarz J, Engelmann K: Cell culture conditions affect RPE phagocytic function. Graefes Arch Clin Exp Ophthalmol 2007;245:981–991.
32 Engelmann K, Friedl P: Growth of human corneal endothelial cells in a serum-reduced medium. Cornea 1995;14:62–70.
33 Engelmann K, Sobottka Ventura A, Drexler D, Staude HJ: A sensitive method for testing the quality of organ culture media and of individual medium components in a cornea bank. Graefes Arch Clin Exp Ophthalmol 1998;236:312–319.
34 Bost LM, Aotaki-Keen AE, Hjelmeland LM: Cellular adhesion regulates bFGF gene expression in human retinal pigment epithelial cells. Exp Eye Res 1994;58:545–552.
35 Campochiaro PA, Sugg R, Grotendorst G, Hjelmeland LM: Retinal pigment epithelial cells produce PDGF-like proteins and secrete them into their media. Exp Eye Res 1989;49:217–227.
36 Esser P, Weller M, Bresgen M, Heimann K, Wiedemann P: The effects of basic fibroblast growth factor on bovine retinal pigment epithelium in vitro. Ger J Ophthalmol 1992;1:58–61.
37 Hackett SF, Schoenfeld CL, Freund J, Gottsch JD, Bhargave S, Campochiaro PA: Neurotrophic factors, cytokines and stress increase expression of basic fibroblast growth factor in retinal pigmented epithelial cells. Exp Eye Res 1997;64:865–873.
38 LaVail MM, Unoki K, Yasumura D, Matthes MT, Yancopoulos GD, Steinberg RH: Multiple growth factors, cytokines, and neurotrophins rescue photoreceptors from the damaging effects of constant light. Proc Natl Acad Sci USA 1992;89:11249–11253.
39 Leschey KH, Hackett SF, Singer JH, Campochiaro PA: Growth factor responsiveness of human retinal pigment epithelial cells. Invest Ophthalmol Vis Sci 1990;31:839–846.
40 Yoshida M, Tanihara H, Yoshimura N: Platelet-derived growth factor gene expression in cultured human retinal pigment epithelial cells. Biochem Biophys Res Commun 1992;189:66–71.
41 Tezel TH, Del Priore LV: Serum-free media for culturing and serial-passaging of adult human retinal pigment epithelium. Exp Eye Res 1998;66:807–815.
42 Bednarz J, Doubilei V, Wollnik PC, Engelmann K: Effect of three different media on serum free culture of donor corneas and isolated human corneal endothelial cells. Br J Ophthalmol 2001;85:1416–1420.
43 Moller-Pedersen T, Hartmann U, Ehlers N, Engelmann K: Evaluation of potential organ culture media for eye banking using a human corneal endothelial cell growth assay. Graefes Arch Clin Exp Ophthalmol 2001;239:778–782.
44 Engelmann K, Valtink M: RPE cell cultivation. Graefes Arch Clin Exp Ophthalmol 2004;242:65–67.
45 Doubilei V, Bednarz J, Valtink M, Zubaty V, Karl MO, Engelmann K, Schäfer H: Serum-free cultivation of adult human retinal pigment epithelial (RPE) cells for transplantation (ARVO abstract 3450). Invest Ophthalmol Vis Sci (Suppl CD-ROM) 2002.

46 Warncke B, Valtink M, Weichel J, Engelmann K, Schaefer H: Experimental rat model for therapeutic retinal pigment epithelium transplantation: unequivocal microscopic identification of human donor cells by in situ hybridisation of human-specific Alu sequences. Virchows Arch 2004;444:74–81.

47 Durlu YK, Tamai M: Transplantation of retinal pigment epithelium using viable cryopreserved cells. Cell Transplant 1997;6:149–162.

48 Valtink M, Engelmann K, Kruger R, Schellhorn ML, Loliger C, Puschel K, Richard G: Structure of a cell bank for transplantation of HLA-typed, cryopreserved human adult retinal pigment epithelial cells (in German). Ophthalmologe 1999;96:648–652.

49 Dunn KC, Aotaki-Keen AE, Putkey FR, Hjelmeland LM: ARPE-19, a human retinal pigment epithelial cell line with differentiated properties. Exp Eye Res 1996;62:155–169.

50 Bednarz J, Teifel M, Friedl P, Engelmann K: Immortalization of human corneal endothelial cells using electroporation protocol optimized for human corneal endothelial and human retinal pigment epithelial cells. Acta Ophthalmol Scand 2000;78:130–136.

Monika Valtink, Dipl.-Ing. (FH) Biotechnologie
Institute of Anatomy
Medical Faculty 'Carl Gustav Carus'
TU Dresden
Fetscherstr. 74
DE–01307 Dresden (Germany)
Tel. +49 0 351 458 6124, Fax +49 0 351 458 6303, E-Mail monika.valtink@tu-dresden.de

Bredehorn-Mayr T, Duncker GIW, Armitage WJ (eds): Eye Banking.
Dev Ophthalmol. Basel, Karger, 2009, vol 43, pp 120–124

Costs and Financing

A Cost Calculation of an Up-to-Date Eye Bank in Germany

D. Böhringer · P. Maier · R. Sundmacher · T. Reinhard

Augenklinik, Universitätsklinikum Freiburg, Freiburg, Deutschland

Abstract

Purpose: To estimate the averaged cost of processing a corneal graft for keratoplasty. **Methods:** We estimated the total running costs of a German corneal bank for one year. All procurement-related expenses were calculated on the basis of 300 donors per year and a disavowal percentage of 50%. **Results:** The running costs comprise of personnel (2 physicians, 2 technicians), amortization of equipment, laboratory costs, laboratory consumables, occupancy costs and quality management. Annual expenses total 584000 EUR. This aggregation divided by 300 corneal grafts released for transplantation results in a nominal charge of 1950 EUR per corneal graft. **Discussion:** The DRG system in Germany (in-patients at a base rate of 1.0) refunds only 850 EUR, leaving a financial gap of 1100 EUR per keratoplasty. This financial burden is currently left over to the eye bank and/or the surgeon.

Graft supply will likely be concentrated in fewer high-volume eye banks due to increasingly stringent national and European regulations [1]. This will result in an overall increase in intercenter graft exchange, necessitating agreement on financial compensation. The graft itself cannot be sold for ethical and legal reasons. However, the financial compensation has to account for both investment and running costs of graft procurement within the eye bank. In this paper, we define these costs from the quota of total eye bank expenses in 1 year by the count of annually transplanted grafts. In order to put this calculation on a firm footing, both investment and running costs from the eye bank have to be considered. This in turn necessitates some economic assumptions as the basis of calculations.

Basis of Calculations

Basic assumptions have to be made about the eye bank and its basic conditions (table 1). All calculations in this chapter assume that corneal grafts are exclusively procured from organ culture.

Table 1. Quantitative assumptions to calculate the annual running costs of a cornea bank in Germany

Entry	Quantity
Donors	300
Corneas	600
Rejection rate, %	50
Grafts	300

Table 2. Basic equipment of a cornea bank – basic investment costs

Amount	Item	Price, EUR
1	microscope	45,000
1	sterile workbench	12,949
3	microcomputers	6,122
2	incubators	11,000
1	slitlamp	5,510
1	sterilizing oven	5,510
2	refrigerators	1,543
Sum		87,634

HLA matching in penetrating keratoplasty is likely to increase in the future due to a mounting body of positive evidence [2]. In order to provide at least high-risk patients with HLA-matched grafts, all donors have to be HLA typed to ensure a sufficiently large pool for HLA matching. The calculation thus includes HLA typing of all donors.

The basic quantitative assumption is an annual rate of 300 quality-controlled corneal grafts issued from the eye bank. This rate is the mean by international standards but reached only by 3 cornea banks in Germany [3]. This rate implies an annual obtainment of 600 corneas from 300 donors assuming a mean rejection rate of 50% due to quality control. The quantitative basis for calculating the running costs is summarized in table 1.

Investment Costs

The basic equipment of a cornea bank comprises at least a sterile workbench, a slitlamp and a phase contrast microscope for quality control, 2 incubators for organ culture (one for sterile grafts, the other for quarantine), 2 refrigerators for culture media and a sterilizing oven for the instruments [1]. Last but not least, workflow and documentation of quality control have to be supported by an electronic data management system. Approximated prices of the basic equipment are listed in table 2. The costs total around EUR 88,000, yielding an annual charge of approximately EUR 18,000 from an estimated annual amortization rate of 20%.

Table 3. Manpower requirements

Job	Occupancy
2 physicians	full time
2 technicians	full time
Data management and software programming	external contractor

Running Costs

Personnel costs are by far the most important contributor to the running costs of a cornea bank. Manpower is required to obtain permission for graft excision from the relatives of the potential donors, to obtain and rate donor information. Tasks specifically requiring a physician include graft assessment and supervision of technicians. Manpower of technicians is required for renewal of organ culture media, data input into the data management system and overall logistics. A database specialist is mandatory for updating the software package, for error recovery and statistical analyses on a regular basis. Table 3 summarizes the manpower required to operate a cornea bank. In order to allow for graft collection on weekends, shift operation and to compensate for vacancies, 2 physicians and technicians each are required (this assumption is based on 30 days of holiday per year, 10 days of educational activities such as conferences or of illness, yielding 220 days a year at work, equalling 8 h of daily working time at 40 h of weekly working time). The costs for physicians comprise one and a half junior interns for routine activities and a half-time senior physician specialized in ophthalmology for supervision and management. The costs for technicians are averaged for age. Personnel costs total around EUR 230,000 a year (table 4).

From the material costs, the most important contributors are laboratory tests followed by commercially available cell culture media. Last but not least, instruments are to be periodically repaired or replaced. Administrative costs comprise office material, public relations activities as well as costs of literature and travel grants. Running costs from material total around EUR 350,000 a year.

Total Costs

The total annual costs of processing 600 grafts add up to EUR 584,000. Due to quality control, only 300 corneas are released for grafting, resulting in a price of EUR 1,950 for a single cornea graft (EUR 584,000/300 released grafts). As running costs are essentially constant over time, the price of a cornea graft is inversely correlated with the rate of released grafts: high-volume eye banks are thus capable of providing grafts at a lower price than smaller ones, processing less than 600 grafts annually. This

Table 4. Calculation of running costs

Running costs	Specification	Price, EUR
Personnel costs	2 technicians 2 physicians	102,200 130,000
Sum		232,200
Consumable material	HLA typings of donors (EUR 600) pharmaceutical products virology/microbiology instrument repair administration	180,000 57,822 40,410 3,500 1,500
Occupancy	rent (100 m^2) cleaning/acclimatization/electricity	24,000 12,000
Amortization	annual rate of 20%	17,527
Certification (ISO)	annual visitation	5,000
Software programming	contractor	10,000
Sum		351,759

dependence of the price of a corneal graft on donor supply places a substantial financial risk on the eye bank administration as overestimation of the donor rate will result in financial losses in 1 year.

Funding

The funding based on diagnosis-related groups for a keratoplasty procedure in Germany (for inpatients at a base rate of 1.0) is calculated to refund the graft at a price of EUR 850. This is far from covering the actual costs of EUR 1,950/graft as calculated above.

Although refunding of procurement costs has substantially improved as of 2007 (previously, only an amount of around EUR 500 was included in the diagnosis-related group calculation), a financial gap of EUR 1,100 remains for each corneal graft. Filling this discrepancy is left to the eye banks and the associated eye hospitals.

Current Situation (as of January 2007)

In general, running costs are not covered by third-party funds. Most costs are rather to be covered by cross-subsidization from budget funds, especially by allocating hospital staff to the eye bank.

On the other hand, investment costs are currently mostly covered by means of third-party funds. Thus, the investment costs of the Lions cornea banks of North-Rhine-Westphalia and of Baden-Württemberg/Regio have mostly been covered by the local Lions clubs and the Lions relief organization. Another common source of funding is the organization DSO-G (Gemeinnützige Gesellschaft für Gewebetransplantation).

The menace of clean-room requirements according to European law could place an additional, substantial economic burden on the German eye banks as the necessary structural modifications are estimated to be as high as EUR 500,000 for most cornea banks. Most of the cornea banks could thus face bankruptcy should these regulations be incorporated into national law.

Outlook

Full cost coverage of corneal grafts should be considered a basic prerequisite of sustained, high-quality graft supply. The funding of the keratoplasty procedure should thus be increased to include all costs associated with graft procurement. A better approach would be direct funding of cornea banks by the healthcare system. This solution could also abolish the unfortunate dependence of the price of a single graft on the unpredictable count of annually obtained corneas, currently imposing the financial risk exclusively on the eye banks.

Additionally, intense networking and political lobbying are currently necessary to prevent the incorporation of the futile clean-room requirements into German law. Partial success has already been achieved by the Arbeitsgemeinschaft Deutscher Hornhautbanken so that this endeavor is considered likely at the time of writing.

References

1 Richtlinien zum Führen einer Hornhautbank. Dtsch Ärztebl 1997;31/32:2122–2124.

2 Böhringer D, Sundmacher R, Reinhard T: Histocompatibility matching in penetrating keratoplasty; in Reinhard T, Larkin F (eds): Cornea and External Eye Disease. Essentials in Ophthalmology. Berlin, Springer, 2006.

3 European Eye Bank Association Directory, ed 15. January 2007.

Dr. Daniel Böhringer
Universitätsaugenklinik Freiburg
Killianstrasse 5
DE–79106 Freiburg (Germany)
Tel. +49 761 270 4001, Fax +49 761 270 4063, E-Mail daniel.boehringer@uniklinik-freiburg.de

Bredehorn-Mayr T, Duncker GIW, Armitage WJ (eds): Eye Banking.
Dev Ophthalmol. Basel, Karger, 2009, vol 43, pp 125–130

Practical Implications of the Law on Tissues for Cornea Banks in Germany[1]

Claudia Hauswald[a] · Timm Bredehorn-Mayr[b]

[a]Interdisciplinary Center for Medicine, Ethics and Law, Martin-Luther-University Halle-Wittenberg, and [b]Eye Clinic, University Hospital of Halle, Halle (Saale), Germany

Abstract

Issue: On August 1, 2007, the Law on the Quality and Safety of Human Tissues and Cells came into force. **Implications:** As a consequence of the new legislation on human tissue, legislative changes were effected upon the Law Regulating Transplantations, Medicine Law and Transfusion Law and the regulation of pharmacies as well as the operating regulations for wholesale pharmaceutical holdings. **Results and Conclusion:** The substantial increase in regulation caused by the Tissue Act far exceeds the requirements of the EC directive on tissues. As such, it has resulted in a huge increase in material (financial, human) and bureaucracy, with no significant gains in safety or quality in an area that had functioned well under the previous legislation.

On August 1, 2007, the Law on the Quality and Safety of Human Tissues and Cells came into force. The Tissue Law in the form of a rule law requires implementing the content of the European Directives 2004/23/EC (Tissue Directive)[2], 2006/86/EC[3] and 2006/17/EC[4]. The Tissue Law necessitates changes to Transplantation Law (TPG,

1 This essay is an abridged version of a thesis as part of the course structure medicine ethics law at the Martin Luther University Halle-Wittenberg, June 2008.

2 Europäisches Parlament und Rat: RL 2004/23/EG vom 31. März 2004 zur Festlegung von Qualitäts- und Sicherheitsstandards für die Spende, Beschaffung, Testung, Verarbeitung, Konservierung, Lagerung und Verteilung von menschlichen Geweben und Zellen. ABl EU L 102 vom 7. April 2004, pp 48ff.

3 Kommission: RL 2006/86/EG vom 24. Oktober 2006 zur Umsetzung der Richtlinie 2004/23/EG hinsichtlich der Anforderungen an die Rückverfolgbarkeit, der Meldung schwerwiegender Zwischenfälle und unerwünschter Reaktionen sowie bestimmter technischer Anforderungen an die Kodierung, Verarbeitung, Konservierung, Lagerung und Verteilung von menschlichen Geweben und Zellen. ABl EU L 294 vom 25. Oktober 2006, pp 32ff.

4 Kommission: RL 2006/17/EG vom 8. Februar 2006 zur Durchführung der Richtlinie 2004/23/EG hinsichtlich technischer Vorschriften für die Spende, Beschaffung und Testung von menschlichen Geweben und Zellen. ABl EU L 38 vom 9. Februar 2006, pp 40ff.

'Transplantationsgesetz'), Medicine Law and Transfusion Law and the regulation of pharmacies as well as the operating regulations for wholesale pharmaceutical holdings. This led to many substantial changes which have to be considered and implemented by German cornea banks.

Legal Situation before Coming into Force of the Tissue Law

Prior to the implementation of the Tissue Law, the TPG[5] from December 1997, as well as the guidelines of the German Medical Association to establish brain death[6] (1997) and for running a cornea bank[7] (August 2000), in conjunction with the detailed provisions of the Association of German Cornea Banks[8] formed the legal framework for cornea banks. This will continue to be the case, albeit in another form in terms of the TPG.

Concrete Effects of the Tissue Act on the Cornea Banks

Drug Law

For the cornea banks the most serious change caused by the Tissue Law is the inclusion of corneas in the Drug Law (AMG, 'Arzneimittelgesetz'). By introducing the concept of 'tissue preparation'[9] in § 4 paragraph 30 AMG, apart from human sperm and ova, all tissues within the meaning of § 1a No. 4 TPG or tissues from such products which produced medicines were elaborated upon. § 1a No. 4 TPG defines tissue as all cells obtained from existing components of the human body which are not defined as organs under No. 1.

The explicit exclusion of corneas from the pharmaceutical term, as it has previously been done in § 2 paragraph 3 No. 8 AMG (old version), has been deleted.

This has far-reaching consequences for the cornea banks.

By widening the scope of corneal tissue, cornea banks will now need a permit for the collection, processing and storage and possibly for the transfer.

There exists a legal distinction between substances found in tissues in the laboratory and research (permit pursuant to § 20b AMG), and those derived from tissue extraction, storage and 'market(ing)' (permit pursuant to § 20c AMG). The latter only applies to those tissues that are not processed industrially, or to those for which the

[5] BGBl 2007;I:1574.
[6] Notice in Dtsch Ärztebl 1998;95:A1861–A1868.
[7] Notice in Dtsch Ärztebl 2000;97:A2122–A2124.
[8] Durchführungsbestimmungen für die Kultivierung von Spenderhornhäuten und die Organisation von Hornhautbanken vom 30. September 2001. www.deutsche-hornhautbanken.de.
[9] The term is considered as a failed manipulation to enable an undifferentiated implementation of the tissue guideline via the Drug Law; see Bundesärztekammer: Stellungnahme zum GewG-E. p. 24.

processing procedure in the EU is well known, for example heart valves, corneas, bone and blood vessels. The permits under §§ 20b and 20c are administered by the material testing board ('Materialprüfungsanstalt') for the establishment of competent national authority. It should be noted that the permission only applies to the specific establishment and specific tissues or laboratories for specific activities, § 20b paragraph 1 p. 5, 20c paragraph 4 p. 3 AMG.

For placement on the market, there is, pursuant to section 21a AMG, a specific authorization issued by the Paul Ehrlich Institute in Langen that is easier to process than the approval for finished products in accordance with § 21 AMG[10]. It pertains mainly to medical and academic material, and clinical trials are not necessary[11].

For all other industrially processed cells and tissues such as hepatocytes or bone tissue, there remains the requirement of obtaining a manufacturing license under § 13 AMG at the national authority and an approval under § 21 AMG at the Paul Ehrlich Institute when requested[12].

Accordingly, there are different sets of requirements necessary for the various licenses and permits that need to be obtained. The requirements for compliance with the principles of 'good practice' (§ 20b AMG) or of 'good manufacturing practice' (§ 13 AMG)[13] being substantially different from one another is a good example of this.

There are also differences in terms of trade in tissue products. For example, the trade in tissues, for the treatment of another person, is banned under § 17 paragraph 1 clause 1 TPG; however, the commercialization of tissue products under the § 21 AMG procedure is allowed, in accordance with § 17 paragraph 1 clause. 2 No. 2 TPG.

In § 63c AMG there are special responsibilities for documentation and reporting of serious incidents or serious adverse reactions for a license holder of tissue preparations pursuant to § 21a AMG.

§ 72b AMG regulates – compared to § 72 AMG – a simplified importation permit from 'well-known' as well as from third countries to Germany[14].

Transplantation Law

The extension of the Law on Tissue Transplants brought about the new § 3a with specific duties of tissue-processing facilities (§ 8d TPG) and higher demands on the laboratory testing of donor tissues (§ 8e TPG). Additionally, in § 8f TPG a registry of

[10] Siegmund-Schultze N: Gewebegesetz: mehr Bürokratie und zu wenig Information. Dtsch Ärztebl 2008;105:A-828.

[11] Pruss A: 4 Fragen an Dr. med. Axel Pruss, Abteilungs- und Herstellungsleiter, Gewebebank der Charité. Dtsch Ärztebl 2007;104:A-1624, B-1436, C-1376.

[12] To the whole: Siegmund-Schultze N: Gewebegesetz: mehr Bürokratie und zu wenig Information. Dtsch Ärztebl 2008;105:A-828.

[13] Parzeller M, Zedler B, Rüdiger C: Das neue Gewebegesetz, iacta alea est. Rechtsmedizin 2007, p 298.

[14] Karbe T, Wulf B, et al: Das neue deutsche Gewebegesetz. Rechtsmedizin 2007, p 382.

tissue establishments has been planned. At this juncture, this registry is only intended to apply to module 1 transplants – and the facilities for tissue acquisition.

§ 1a No. 8 TPG legally defines the 'tissue establishment' as a body that extracts, investigates, processes, treats, preserves, marks, packages or delivers tissue for the purpose of transfer to somebody.

A cornea bank, which removes and investigates tissue, may only be operated under § 8d paragraph 1 clause 1 TPG regardless of pharmaceutical regulatory requirements if technical qualification and expertise are guaranteed by a doctor.

The rule also contains specific requirements for compliance with the state of medical science and technology for the removal, the donor medical evaluation and laboratory tests required for processing, manufacturing, preservation and storage of tissues[15]. The details pursuant to § 8d paragraph 1 clause 3 TPG constitute a legal regulation under § 16a. In that regard, as from the beginning of April 2008, the implementation of the TPG tissue regulation[16] from March 26, 2008, has to be observed.

§ 8d paragraph 2 includes extensive documentation requirements. Accordingly, a tissue institution needs to document every tissue removal and delivery as well as the related measures and available details with regard to its application in products and materials for purposes of e.g. transparency, risk monitoring or tracking.

These documents must be kept, for the purpose of tracing, for at least 30 years after the end of the tissue expiration date according to § 15 paragraph 2 TPG.

In addition to this, every tissue institution must document and make information on their activities publically available. This includes the details about the nature and quantity of the collected/analyzed/processed/treated or processed/preserved/stored/delivered or otherwise used, imported or exported tissues. This is made in the form of submitting an annual report[17] to the federal authority and the Paul Ehrlich Institute, according to § 8 paragraph 3 TPG.

Such a scheme provides clear benefits. It results in improved transparency in connection with the report of the federal government which is issued every 4 years with regard to the supply of the population with tissues and tissue preparations under article 7a Tissue Law which allows for a good overview as to which tissues are available and to what extent.

This may for example be compared with the Federal Ministry of Health's repeated demands for an allocation guideline on the lack of tissues as a response to potential shortfalls in supply. Surely, such a comprehensive documentation requirement on the tissue establishments would also strengthen the confidence of the general population in what has been a relatively neglected area. On the other hand, it means an enormous

[15] Parzeller M, Zedler B, Rüdiger C: Das neue Gewebegesetz, iacta alea est. Rechtsmedizin 2007, p 296.

[16] Verordnung über die Anforderungen an Qualität und Sicherheit der Entnahme von Geweben und deren Übertragung nach dem Transplantationsgesetz vom 26. März 2008. BGBl 2008;I:512ff.

[17] Available on the homepage of the Paul Ehrlich Institute: www.pei.de.

increase in administrative work for the tissue banks and consequently a need for additional staff.

Pursuant to § 8e TPG, laboratory tests for tissue donors may only be carried out in a research laboratory that is accredited in accordance with the requirements of the AMG and accordingly achieve additional quality assurance measures.

§ 13c TPG requires tissue establishments to lay down a specific tracing procedure for tissue leading to serious incidents[18] or serious adverse reactions[19].

Pharmaceutical Ingredient Production Regulation

A subordination of corneas under the medicines term also requires that the cornea banks must now observe the Pharmaceutical Ingredient Production Regulation[20]. By amending the provisions of the Pharmaceutical Ingredient Production Regulation of March 26, 2008[21], its scope has been explicitly expanded on facilities, i.e. the tissues which are – pursuant to § 1a No. 4 TPG – commercially produced, tested, stored, placed etc. In this context, the new requirements of the redrafted § 5a bring into force new special rules for collection, tissue establishments and tissue donors for laboratories.

Conclusion

The substantial increase in regulation caused by the Tissue Act far exceeds the requirements of the EC directive on tissues. As such, this has resulted in a huge increase in material (financial, human) and bureaucracy, with no significant gains in safety or quality in an area that had functioned well under the previous legislation.

Whether all this actually results in an improvement in the supply of tissues can only be assessed when the first report by the Federal Government under Article 7a Tissue Law will be issued in 2010.

18 Legally defined in § 1a No. 10 TPG as any untoward event in connection with the collection, analysis, processing, manufacturing or processing or distribution of tissues, the transmission of a contagious illness, death or a life-threatening condition, a disability or a loss of ability of patients, which may result in or require hospitalization, prolong an illness or renew such intrusions.

19 Legally defined in § 1a No. 11 TPG as an unintended response, including a transmissible disease, by the donor or recipient to the removal or transfer of tissues, which is fatal or life-threatening, which gives rise to a disability or loss of ability, which requires hospitalization or prolongs a hospital stay, or which leads to a disease or prolongs it.

20 Verordnung über die Anwendung der Guten Herstellungspraxis bei der Herstellung von Arzneimitteln und Wirkstoffen und über die Anwendung der Guten Fachlichen Praxis bei der Herstellung von Produkten menschlicher Herkunft vom 3. November 2006. BGBl 2006;I:2523ff.

21 Notice in BGBl 2008;I:521ff.

Acknowledgement

Translation support by Kevin Koh and Philipp Skarupinski.

Further Reading

Arbeitsgruppe Hornhautspende, -banking und -verteilung in Deutschland: Spende, Banking und Verteilung von Augenhornhäuten – eine bundesweite Befragung von Banken und Transplanteuren. 2004. www.gewebenetzwerk.de/docman/allgemein/bedarfsstudie-hornhaut/download.html.

Bender AW: Organtransplantation und AMG. VersR 1999, pp 419ff.

Bundesärztekammer: Eckpunktepapier 'Zellen und Gewebe' vom 15. April 2005. www.bäk.de.

Bundesärztekammer: Erweiterte und aktualisierte Stellungnahme zum Regierungsentwurf für ein Gewebegesetz vom 24. Januar 2007. www.bäk.de.

Herrig C: Die Gewebetransplantation nach dem Transplantationsgesetz: Entnahme–Lagerung–Verwendung unter besonderer Berücksichtigung der Hornhauttransplantation. Frankfurt am Main, Lang, 2002.

Karbe T, Wulf B, Jakob S, Heinemann A, Kammal M, Püschel K, Montenero M, Parzeller M: Das neue deutsche Gewebegesetz unter Berücksichtigung des TPG-Gewebeverordnungsentwurfs hinsichtlich praktischer Umsetzung der postmortalen Gewebespende. Rechtsmedizin 2007, pp 380ff.

Parzeller M, Zedler B, Rüdiger C: Das neue Gewebegesetz, iacta alea est. Rechtsmedizin 2007, pp 293ff.

Pruss A: 4 Fragen an Dr. med. Axel Pruss, Abteilungs- und Herstellungsleiter, Gewebebank der Charité. Dtsch Ärztebl 2007;104:A-1624, B-1436, C-1376.

Siegmund-Schultze N: Gewebegesetz: mehr Bürokratie und zu wenig Information. Dtsch Ärztebl 2008;105: A-828.

Wilhelm FW, Duncker GIW, Bredehorn T (eds): Augenbanken. Berlin, de Gruyter, 2002.

T. Bredehorn-Mayr
Eye Clinic, University Hospital of Halle (Saale)
DE–06120 Halle (Saale) (Germany)
Tel. +49 345 5571878, Fax +49 345 5571848, E-Mail timm.bredehorn@medizin.uni-halle.de

Bredehorn-Mayr T, Duncker GIW, Armitage WJ (eds): Eye Banking.
Dev Ophthalmol. Basel, Karger, 2009, vol 43, pp 131–135

European Association of Tissue Banks

Michael Cahane[a] · Jeroen van Baare[b]

[a]EATB Ocular Council and Sheba Medical Center Eye Bank Tel Hashomer, Tel Hashomer, Israel; [b]Tissue Services Europe and Medical Innovations, Best, The Netherlands

Abstract

Tissue banking is a specific field of medical practice. The European Association of Tissue Banks (EATB) is a scientific nonprofit organization that coordinates and supports aspects of tissue banking within Europe. The evolvement, structure and principal fields of interest and activities of the EATB are described.

Tissue for transplantation includes bone, skin, heart valves, corneas and other tissues as well.

The need for human tissue for transplantation dates back a long time in history and is already expressed in a legendary story from the 6th century in which Saints Cosmas and Damian successfully transplanted a limb. The massive bone allograft was taken from a Moor who had died earlier that morning [1].

The Dutch surgeon Job Van Meekren was the first to document the use of a bone graft in 1668. He used a piece of canine skull to replace a skull defect in a Russian nobleman. Although a successful operation, it resulted in the patient's excommunication by the church [2]. The first skin transplant was reported in 1869 [3], and in 1905 Edward Zirm performed the first corneal transplantation [4].

The modern practice of tissue banking started in the 20th century. The first tissue bank in Europe was established in Czechoslovakia in 1952, retrieving corneas, skin and bones [5].

Since that day, new techniques (cryopreservation, freeze-drying) for long-term preservation have been developed, and tissues became available for many patients.

Improved techniques for processing and preservation are now allowing for the use of more specific treatment for a wide variety of tissue defects. In the last 5 decades, tissue allografts became an important surgical tool, significantly enhancing the quality of human life, and even life saving.

The use of human allograft tissues for surgery has proven that the use of a safe and of a high-quality allograft tissue is essential for complete and successful treatment [6].

Relevant issues of importance include not only the structural quality of the allograft tissue, but also bacteriological and serological safety, for the protection of the recipient (as well as the tissue banking staff) from transmissible diseases.

Tissue banks began introducing technical and medical standards in order to ensure the highest quality and safety of allograft tissues. Subsequently national governments recognized the importance of establishing general standards which also include ethical issues concerning tissue banking. National regulations were gradually introduced, and tissue banking developed into a very specific field of medical practice.

As the demand for allograft tissues increased, and usually exceeded the supply, the need for international cooperation between tissue banks for the exchange of tissues became apparent. The American Association of Tissue Banks was founded in 1976. Europe followed by the establishment of the European Association of Tissue Banks (EATB) in 1991 as the European platform for the exchange of ideas on all aspects of tissue banking.

Organization

The EATB is a scientific, nonprofit organization that coordinates and promotes all aspects of tissue banking within Europe. It supports cooperation between tissue banks in the fields of research and development, and facilitates the availability and exchange of transplantable tissues and cells with the highest quality to meet the national and European demands and standards.

The association publishes its own standards to ensure that the conduct of tissue banking meets acceptable norms of technical and ethical performance. These standards relate to donation, procurement, processing, preservation and distribution of transplantable tissue. Specifics include donor selection criteria, necessary testing (including screening for HIV and hepatitis), maintenance of asepsis, labeling, storage, distribution and record keeping.

The EATB also supports programs for training, accreditation and certification of tissue bank personnel to ensure that banking activities are performed in a professional manner.

In its effort to keep tissue banking at the highest quality level, the EATB maintains close liaisons with official health-related institutions in all European states and with the European Union, engaging in an ongoing program of information exchange.

The EATB website can be found on www.eatb.de (to be changed soon to www.eatb.eu).

Standards

In its early years, the EATB's most important mission was the establishment and distribution of standards. Previously, each member state had its own laws and standards. The goal was to recommend a common set of minimal standards based on scientific and medical knowledge that could be implemented by all European tissue banks. In each and every field of tissue banking, the EATB set performance requirements intended to prevent disease transmission as well as ensure optimal clinical performance of transplanted tissues and cells.

EATB and European Union

In an attempt to increase harmonization and regulation in the European Community, a directive for tissue banking was introduced by the European Council in March 2004 [7]. The EATB was an actively involved partner in the development of this directive which EU membership states are obliged to adopt and implement (in addition to other directives that will affect tissue banking). A new directive for tissue engineering is currently being proposed. This may have a major impact on tissue banking in Europe. The EATB is also involved in these discussions, in an attempt to influence future legislation in such a way that it will protect as well as encourage tissue banking activities. Although regulation and harmonization are both noteworthy and desirable goals, they should not become overly restrictive as it may lower the availability of tissues for transplantation.

Education and Cooperation with Other Organizations

The EATB provides a scientific forum for the exchange of information by holding conferences and promoting practical courses and workshops. It publishes proceedings from these meetings, newsletters and other educational material relevant to tissue banking. It supports research and coordinates international study groups.

The Association maintains cooperative programs with other scientific and professional organizations throughout the world to keep its members informed about the latest medical applications of preserved allografts and to assess their clinical efficacy. Consequently, the most updated information regarding new developments in tissue banking is available to each and every member.

The Association is also designed to serve as a source of information and advice to individuals and organizations wishing to establish or expand banking activities.

The EATB is working closely together with the American Association of Tissue Banks, Latin American Association of Tissue Banks and the Asian Pacific Association of Tissue Banks.

EATB and Eye Banking Activities

The EATB Ocular Council is one of the councils founded within the Association. Its early mission was to formulate the minimal standards for eye banking. At the same time the Ocular Council and EATB began to work in close cooperation with the European Eye Bank Association (EEBA). As regulation in Europe seemed to increase and the formulation of new laws and directives was bound to appear, ties between EATB and EEBA became a necessity. Both organizations realized that in order to influence new laws and regulation, eye banking standards should be represented in a harmonious manner. For that reason, an EATB representative was also invited to attend the EEBA committee meetings.

This partnership led to the creation of eye banking standards that were acceptable for both organizations. Adoption of the same minimal standards led to the creation of one system of rules and standards over Europe, and it could be adopted by eye banks and tissue banks on a voluntary basis (before the EC directives were published).

Since eye banking is one of the areas of tissue banking that is included in the EC directive, although it has its own distinctive features, both associations could now have the same attitude and a single voice while trying to influence the new regulatory rules and directives.

Regulation has also economical aspects. Regulation in Europe may lead to the closure of small eye banks that will not be able to meet the higher performance standards. Some tissue banks are already practicing eye banking as part of the tissue banking activities. The practice of tissue banking (and eye banking) becomes more professional. Regulation will make it hard to procure and process tissues (including corneas) in small hospitals that have no tissue or cornea banks. For those reasons, the EATB predicts that in the near future it might be expected that more eye banking activities will be incorporated into tissue banks.

Councils and Committees

In order to achieve the aims of the Association, councils and committees are established in order to share the expertise of a large variety of tissue banks and to come to harmonized standards.

Current councils include:
- Musculoskeletal
- Skin
- Heart valve
- Ocular
- Reproductive
- Tissue banking (general)

Committees include:

- Standards
- Ethics and legal
- Education
- Finance
- Scientific
- Accreditation and membership

Membership

EATB membership might be on an individual or institutional basis. Individual membership is offered to those who are involved or interested in banking of tissues, cells or organs, and who concur with and support the objectives, policies and ethical standards set forth by the Association. Individual members receive reduced member rates for EATB meetings. EATB newsletter, membership directory and other publications are included in annual membership dues. Individual members have full voting privileges.

Institutional membership is open to organizations qualifying as accredited full-service tissue banking, including procurement, processing, storage and distribution in accordance with the objectives, policies and ethical standards of the Association. Each institutional member can have 2 representatives for voting.

References

1 Rinaldi E: The first homoplastic limb transplant according to the legend of Saint Cosmas and Saint Damian. Ital J Orthop Traumatol 1987;13:394–406.

2 de Boer H: The history of bone grafts. Clin Orthop 1988;226:292–298.

3 Chick LR: Brief history and biology of skin grafting. Ann Plast Surg 1988;21:358–365.

4 Moffatt SL, Cartwright VA, Stumpf TH: Centennial review of corneal transplantation. Clin Exp Ophthalmol 2005;33:642–657.

5 Mika P: Brief history of the tissue bank, Charles University Hospital, Hradec Kralové, Czech Republic. Cell Tissue Banking 2000;1:17–25.

6 Eastlund T: Infectious disease transmission through tissue transplantation. Adv Tissue Banking 2003;7:51–131.

7 Directive 2004/23/EC on setting standards of quality and safety for the donation, procurement, testing, processing, preservation, storage and distribution of human tissues and cells. Official Journal of the European Union, L102/48, 7 April 2004.

Michael Cahane, MD
EATB Ocular Council and Sheba Medical Center Eye Bank
Tel Hashomer 52621 (Israel)
Tel./Fax +972 3 6295228, E-Mail cahane@netvision.net.il

Author Index

Subject Index